Advancements in Digital Health and Care

Stefanie Scholz • Marion Wüchner-Fuchs
Kurt Höller
Editors

Advancements in Digital Health and Care

Empowering Healthcare Through Innovation, Strategies and Ethical Considerations

Springer

Editors
Stefanie Scholz
Faculty of Engineering
Ansbach University of Applied Sciences
Ansbach, Bayern, Germany

Marion Wüchner-Fuchs
Department of Health, Education
and Sciences
SRH University Heidelberg, Campus Fürth
Fürth, Germany

Kurt Höller
Healthcare Vertical Market
Siemens AG
Erlangen, Germany

ISBN 978-3-032-16836-8 ISBN 978-3-032-16837-5 (eBook)
https://doi.org/10.1007/978-3-032-16837-5

This work was supported by SRH Hochschulen GmbH.

This Springer imprint is published by the registered company Springer Nature Switzerland AG
The registered company address is: Gewerbestrasse 11, 6330 Cham, Switzerland

Foreword

Bavarian State Minister of Health, Care and Prevention

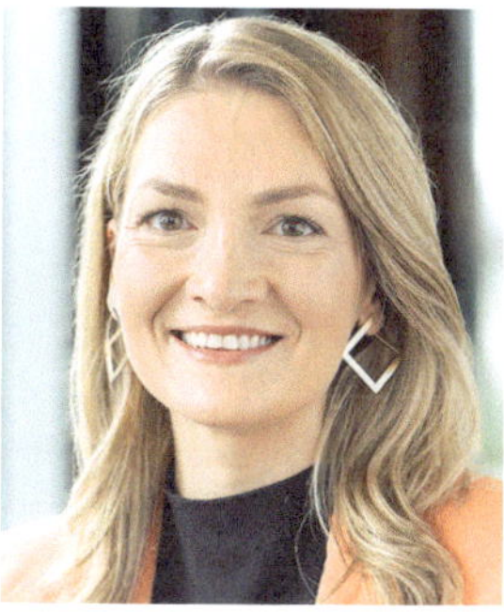

Source: Picture by Bavarian State Ministry of Health, Care and Prevention

Dear Readers,

Digitalisation has revolutionised healthcare fundamentally. Innovations and advances in technology have paved the way for new approaches to patient-centred, efficient, and networked services. The implementation of digital strategies into practice has become a key plank in the context of increasing demands on quality, accessibility, and sustainability.

This publication addresses therefore the "Advancements in Digital Health and Care" as the driver of change in the healthcare sector. It brings together the voices of decision-makers from healthcare providers, payers, and researchers, reflecting on both the opportunities and the challenges of digital transformation. It will present not only strategic views and theoretical foundations but also concrete experiences and practical lessons learnt. Best-practice approaches as well as important insights gained from challenging implementation processes will be highlighted.

The topic comprises a broad spectrum. It provides a baseline overview on technological and ethical dimensions of digital health. It covers data protection, transparency, and the responsible use of sensitive health data. Furthermore included are regulatory frameworks and strategic questions regarding sustainable implementation in clinical, outpatient, and long-term care structures. It also examines patient-centred approaches, the perspectives of healthcare payers, and the issues of equal opportunities and inclusion. Rather than widening the "Digital Divide" and disadvantaging vulnerable social groups, digitalisation of healthcare should instead enhance chances for greater health equity. Only a comprehensive approach taking equal account of technology, strategies, and ethics can really unfold the full potential of digital transformation.

Together, let's unlock change in the healthcare sector, seize its opportunities, and tackle its challenges responsibly. This publication shall guide you in this endeavour and provide impetus for intensive dialogues and sustainable progress. The future of healthcare starts right now, and we can shape it—innovatively, strategically, and ethically well-founded.

All the best

Bavarian State Minister
of Health, Care and Prevention
Munich, Germany

Judith Gerlach

Contents

About the Editors

Stefanie Scholz is a Professor of Data Science at the Faculty of Engineering at Ansbach University of Applied Sciences. Her research focuses on digital health and the application of AI-driven data analytics to improve healthcare delivery and patient outcomes. She is particularly interested in fostering patient empowerment and optimizing intersectoral care processes through digital transformation and user-centered design. In addition to her academic role, Prof. Dr. Scholz has been a member of the expert pool of the Innovation Committee of the Federal Joint Committee (Gemeinsamer Bundesausschuss, G-BA) since 2020, where she contributes her expertise to the evaluation and advancement of innovative healthcare concepts in Germany.

Marion Wüchner-Fuchs is a professor of Social Pedagogy. One of her areas of specialization is the digital empowerment of people with disabilities, as well as the use of digital technologies to enhance accessibility. Her research integrates technological, social, and pedagogical perspectives to promote equitable participation and inclusive learning environments.

Kurt Höller acts as Senior Director of Digital Affairs within the Healthcare Vertical Market team at Siemens AG. His industry development role embraces various aspects of digitalization and sustainability transformation for smart hospitals.

Part I

Introduction to Digital Health and Care

Evolution of Digital Technologies in Healthcare

1

Sara Perez Guzman and Dani Sharl Ajami

1.1 Introduction to Digital Health and Care

1.1.1 Overview of Key Historical Milestones in Digital Health in Germany

A series of legal, institutional, and technological advancements over the past decade has significantly influenced Germany's evolution in digital health. A major milestone in this journey was the enactment of the E-Health Act ("E-Health-Gesetz") in 2015, which established a comprehensive framework for digital infrastructure and mandated the creation of the telematics infrastructure ("Telematik-Infrastruktur," TI), the national digital health backbone of Germany [1]. In practice, this law enabled services such as the e-prescription (eRezept), which by 2022 had connected over 99% of pharmacies to the TI [2] and introduced reimbursement for teleconsultations, allowing general practitioners and psychotherapists to provide video visits covered by statutory insurance, which is a service that became especially important during the COVID 19 pandemic [3]. This legislative framework provided the groundwork for secure data exchange between healthcare providers and insurers, thereby enhancing the integration of digital health services. Later legislation, including the Digital Health Care Act [4] and the Hospital Future Act [5], further expanded access to digital healthcare and introduced incentives for the modernization of healthcare facilities.

One noticeable development in the healthcare sector has been the implementation of the electronic patient record ("elektronische Patientenakte", ePA), which was launched in 2021. The digital patient records are designed to help with medical documents, medication plans, and discharge summaries, thereby improving

S. Perez Guzman (✉) · D. S. Ajami
Department of Health, Education and Social Sciences, SRH University of Applied Sciences, Campus Fuerth, Fürth, Germany
e-mail: Sara.PerezGuzman@stud.srh-university.de; DaniSharl.Ajami@stud.srh-university.de

S. Scholz et al. (eds.), *Advancements in Digital Health and Care*,
https://doi.org/10.1007/978-3-032-16837-5_1

communication across various healthcare sectors [6]. Despite its potential benefits, adoption rates remain relatively low; as of the end of 2023, only 6–16% of insured individuals are using ePA [7]. By contrast, countries such as Finland have achieved much higher levels of adaptation: the "My Kanta patient portal," integrated into Finland's national EHR system, is actively used by more than 90% of citizens to access prescriptions and medical records [8]. This gap illustrates that while Germany has invested in technical infrastructure and patient engagement, trust remains a substantial barrier compared to frontrunners in Northern Europe. Several barriers contribute to this lack of uptake, including inadequate public awareness, concerns regarding privacy, and insufficient guidance from healthcare professionals during the onboarding process [9]. In response to these challenges, the Gesundheitsdatennutzungsgesetz (GDNG) will introduce an opt-out model beginning in 2025, which will automatically enroll all insured individuals unless they explicitly object.

The COVID-19 pandemic influenced significant advancements in the realm of telemedicine. Surveys indicated that more than 50% of outpatient physicians transitioned to video or telephone consultation, with the highest uptake in general practice and mental health, where remote psychotherapy and cognitive behavioral therapy proved effective in maintaining consistent care for patients with depression and anxiety disorders [3, 10]. By contrast, adoption was markedly lower in chronic disease management, such as cardiology and diabetes care, where the need for physical examinations and long-term monitoring limited the effectiveness of virtual visits [3].

Institutions such as Zentrum für Telemedizin (ZTM) in Bad Kissingen, established in 2010, expanded their services on a national scale, facilitating remote diagnostics and chronic care monitoring [11]. Nonetheless, persistent structural disparities between medical specialties and inconsistent broadband access continue to pose challenges to comprehensive integration of telemedicine across healthcare systems [2].

TI has experienced extensive implementation across the healthcare system; by 2022, it was reported that over 99% of pharmacies and 96% of outpatient clinics had established connectivity [2]. This initiative, supported by nearly 774 million euros in funding from statutory health insurers, is designed to facilitate secure communication and provide essential services, including electronic prescriptions and the integration of Digital Health Applications (DiGA) [2]. Nevertheless, TI has encountered significant criticism regarding its frequent technical downtimes and the complexities associated with the user authentication process. In response to these challenges, the development of TI 2.0, which is a streamlined application-based redesign, has been initiated, with efforts underway since 2023 [12].

1.1.2 From Digitalizing to Digital Transformation in Germany

Digitalization initiatives have predominantly focused on comprehensive efforts to transform analog systems into digital formats, manifesting in endeavors such as the implementation of EHRs and the development of robust data infrastructures. In contrast, digital transformation requires a greater focus on reconfiguring care delivery, organizational structures, and the overall patient experiences. The healthcare system in Germany, which is known for its decentralized governance and its strong cultural emphasis on data privacy, has realized significant technical advancements. However, it continues with substantial cultural and institutional resistance that obstructs the pursuit of more comprehensive reforms.

A clearer example of transformation, beyond digitalization, is Germany's reimbursement of remote patient monitoring (RPM) for heart failure, effective since January 2022. This program enables coordinated care across cardiologists, general practitioners, and telemedical centers, with patients reporting daily vital signs, such as weight, blood pressure, and ECG, to central telemedical units that can trigger early interventions, thus reorganizing care rather than merely digitizing records [13]. Similarly, AI-driven triage systems in emergency departments have demonstrated the ability to prioritize patients based on clinical urgency, leading to improved workflow efficiency and significantly reduced waiting times. Real-world applications reported reductions of up to 30% in average patient wait times following the integration of AI-supported triage systems [14]. These cases show that while digitization lays the groundwork, true transformation arises when digital solutions are integrated into new models of care delivery and decision-making processes.

Programs like the KHZG provided over 4.3 billion euros to fund hospitals' IT upgrades and improve digital maturity [15]. The DigitalRadar Hospital Survey revealed that while some hospitals have implemented foundational digital capabilities, significant development requirements remain in areas such as structured data use, interoperability, and patient-centered digital services [15]. Moreover, many facilities still lack qualified IT staff, digital leadership, and effective use of new tools [2].

Cultural resistance has a significant influence on the adaptation and effectiveness of digital health tools. Studies indicate that trust in digital tools depends strongly on usability, data transparency, and the involvement of healthcare professionals. Supporting patients, particularly those with low digital literacy, is essential to ensure effective adoption [9]. Notably, over 50% of patients report feeling inadequately informed about the ePA. Also, a substantial portion expressed a preference for explanations that are delivered by healthcare providers rather than relying on self-directed learning [7]. Among healthcare providers, obstacles to effective implementation include insufficient training, time constraints, and difficulties with the integration of digital tools with existing administrative burdens [16].

Emerging opportunities in the field of health data utilization are becoming increasingly evident. The General Data Protection Regulation (GDPR) and the Artificial Intelligence (AI) Act facilitate the structured secondary use of health data for research purposes, while simultaneously ensuring compliance with GDPR guidelines. Additionally, approved DiGAs, which are regulated by the Federal Institute for Drugs and Medical Devices (BfArM), empower patients to manage chronic conditions such as depression, diabetes, and back pain. By 2025, it is projected that over 50 DiGA applications will be approved (a complete and up-to-date approved DiGA can be accessed on the official website of BfArM).

Concrete clinical examples already demonstrate their potential and how DiGA application can provide multiple health benefits and improved outcomes. The DiGA "Deprexis," an app-based cognitive-behavioral therapy tool for depression, has been tested in randomized controlled trials and shown to significantly reduce depressive symptoms as measured by the PHQ-9 compared with control groups [17]. Moreover, other internet-based CBT interventions have reported meaningful symptom reductions, more than a 50% decrease in PHQ-score, which was relative to control groups [18].

Furthermore, the musculoskeletal therapy app VIVRA is a DiGA application designed to provide individualized exercise programs. Clinical studies have demonstrated that after 12 weeks of use, the app can lead to significant reductions in back pain intensity and improvements in spinal mobility among patients with axial spondylarthritis [19].

The integration of wearable devices, patient portals, and structured EHR data could strongly influence the improvement of data-driven care; however, challenges persist in this particular domain. Major obstacles include problems related to technical interoperability, the development of effective data governance frameworks, and the necessity for explainable AI that can foster trust among both physicians and patients [20]. As digital transformation initiatives progress in Germany, it will be imperative to not only sustain financial investment but also promote a paradigm shift toward co-design methodologies, interdisciplinary collaboration, and innovation that prioritizes patient-centered approaches.

1.1.3 The Digital Transformation of Healthcare: Milestones, Catalysts, and Challenges

The digital revolution in healthcare is fundamentally reshaping the perspective of care services, supported by the development of concepts and innovative technologies. The World Health Organization (WHO) provides valuable terminology to navigate this broad field. The journey initiates with eHealth, which can be defined as the utilization of information and communication technology (ICT) to support healthcare and related fields. This concept includes a wide spectrum of applications, from the implementation of early EHRs to the rise of remote consultations.

Based on this fundamental model, more specific applications have emerged. mHealth (mobile health) constitutes a subcategory of eHealth (electronic health), supported by mobile technologies and smartphones with the aim of delivering healthcare services and sharing health information directly to the patients. Simultaneously, Telehealth utilizes telecommunications and virtual technologies to provide medical care outside traditional clinical environments, therefore closing geographic barriers and enhancing access to healthcare services [21]. Nowadays, these developments are part of the extensive umbrella of digital health, which also includes the usage of advanced domains such as big data analytics, genomics, machine learning, deep learning, and AI. This revolution represents a transition from simple digitization toward a new era characterized by personalized, predictive, and engaging medicine.

The healthcare transformation is followed by multiple technological achievements. Among the most utilized tools is the e-prescription (Electronic Prescription), which, facilitated by governmental initiatives, has established a full integration with the EHR systems, including for controlled substances, has had a positive impact streamlining essential workflows for all healthcare workers [22]. Furthermore, the ability to enhance patients' access to their EHR empowers them to take a more proactive role in their healthcare. Digital tools, including patient portals, mobile applications, and wearable devices, provide patients with direct access to their health data, fostering engagement and enabling informed decision-making. This evolution is key to improving personalized medicine, which seeks to build specific treatments based on the previous patient's data collected from different sources.

Nevertheless, the biggest challenge, in terms of a fully data-driven ecosystem depends on interoperability, which translates to the capacity of multiple systems to be able to seamlessly exchange, interpret, and utilize clinical and medical data. Despite progress in this field, there are still multiple challenges. Many healthcare organizations continue to rely on the regulatory aspect of the systems in charge of generating the data repositories, indirectly blocking the information sharing processes [23]. Moreover, the high costs associated with oversaturated systems, combined with strict data privacy and security regulations such as the GDPR in the European Union or Health Insurance Portability and Accountability Act (HIPAA), add additional challenges to achieve this goal [24]. A deeper challenge arises from the FHIR puzzle (Fast Healthcare Interoperability Resources). While the FHIR standard facilitates data exchange, it does not guarantee a standardization protocol. Consequently, data originating from unrelated EHRs may not be easily comprehended without considerable manual intervention, as variations in coding and terminology delay the analysis necessary for advanced AI applications [25].

1.1.4 The COVID-19 Pandemic: A Catalyst for Unprecedented Adoption

Although the digital evolution of healthcare has been in progress for an extended period, the COVID-19 pandemic acted as a powerful, unanticipated catalyst, compressing a decade's worth of digital acceptance into mere months. The global health crisis exerted immense pressure on healthcare systems around the world, disrupting routine in-person care and precipitating an urgent need for remote solutions [26].

During the pandemic, telehealth transformed from an emerging service into a fundamental component of healthcare services. Adoption rates also improved; by April 2020, most countries had adopted telemedicine as a substitute for face-to-face consultations. In countries such as the United Kingdom and the Netherlands, 64–80% of primary care providers transitioned to telemedicine consultation. In France, the volume of reimbursed teleconsultations increased more than ten times within a single week. For many patients, this represented their initial experience with virtual care; recent research based on COVID-19 pandemic insights and lessons learned showed that 84% of patients utilizing telehealth in March 2020 had never engaged with it before, compared to nowadays [27].

This quick change led to long-term improvements in the healthcare system. Regulatory bodies quickly adjusted their regulations by adopting emergency measures that made the telehealth reimbursement and practices permanent. For example, in Norway, a temporary law that allowed e-consultations to issue sick leave certificates became a permanent measure in 2023 after it proved effective during the pandemic [21]. This large-scale deployment served as a significant proof of concept, overcoming years of clinical research and familiarizing millions with remote care modalities. The pandemic effectively eliminated traditional alternatives to in-person care, demonstrating that necessity can significantly excel innovation-driven adoption of new technologies. While the mentioned achievements highlight the Digital Health improvement, there is still an ongoing debate about the long-term viability of payment and reimbursement, as well new emerging challenges of digital equity leaving an uncertain implementation landscape [28]. The pandemic, therefore, did not create specifically a digital future but rather raised the baseline expectation for it, shifting the discussion from whether digital health will be essential to the modalities by which it will be integrated and optimized for a more resilient healthcare system [27].

References

1. BMG. 2015. E-Health-Gesetz. Available from: https://www.bundesgesundheitsministerium.de/service/gesetze-und-verordnungen/detail/e-health-gesetz.html .
2. McKinsey & Company. German e-health offerings expand, but adoption remains uneven. 2022 [cited 2025 Aug 7]. Available from: https://www.mckinsey.com/industries/life-sciences/our-insights/german-e-healthofferings-expand-but-adoption-remains-uneven#/.
3. Knörr V, Dini L, Gunkel S, Hoffmann J, Mause L, Ohnhäuser T, et al. Use of telemedicine in the outpatient sector during the COVID-19 pandemic: a cross-sectional survey of German physicians. BMC Prim Care. 2022;23(1):92.
4. Gesetz für sichere digitale Kommunikation und Anwendungen im Gesundheitswesen sowie zur Änderung weiterer Gesetze. Bundesgesetzblatt Teil I. 2015 Dec 28;(54):2408.
5. BMG. 2024. Krankenhauszukunftsgesetz (KHZG). Available from: https://www.bundesgesundheitsministerium.de/krankenhauszukunftsgesetz.html. [cited 2025 Aug 5]
6. Rau E, Tischendorf T, Mitzscherlich B. Implementation of the electronic health record in the German healthcare system: an assessment of the current status and future development perspectives considering the potentials of health data utilisation by representatives of different stakeholder groups. Front Health Serv. 2024;4:1370759.
7. Kröner S, Schreiweis B, Strotbaum V, Brandl LC, Pobiruchin M, Wiesner M. Consumer perspectives on the national electronic health record and barriers to its adoption in Germany: does health policy require a change in communication? BMC Health Serv Res. 2025;25(1):33.
8. Jormanainen V, Lindgren M, Keskimäki I, Kaila M. Use of my Kanta in Finland 2010–2022. Stud Health Technol Inform. 2023;305:448–51.
9. von Kalckreuth N, Kopka M, Schmid C, Kratzer C, Reptuschenko A, Feufel MA. Trustworthiness of the electronic health record in Germany: an exploratory, user-centered analysis. Front Digit Health. 2025 Mar 7 [cited 2025 Aug 5]. Available from: https://www.frontiersin.org/journals/digitalhealth/articles/10.3389/fdgth.2025.1473326/full.

10. Peine A, Paffenholz P, Martin L, Dohmen S, Marx G, Loosen SH. Telemedicine in Germany during the COVID-19 pandemic: multi-professional national survey. J Med Internet Res. 2020;22(8):e19745.
11. Center for Telemedicine. In: Wikipedia. 2025 [cited 2025 Aug 7]. Available from: https://en.wikipedia.org/w/index.php?title=Center_for_Telemedicine&oldid=1304412415.
12. TI 2.0 | gematik. [cited 2025 Aug 7]. Available from: https://www.gematik.de/telematikinfrastruktur/ti-2-0
13. Koehler F, Störk S, Schulz M. Telemonitoring of heart failure patients is reimbursed in Germany: challenges of real-world implementation remain. Eur Heart J Digit Health. 2022;3(2):121–2.
14. Da'Costa A, Teke J, Origbo JE, Osonuga A, Egbon E, Olawade DB. AI-driven triage in emergency departments: a review of benefits, challenges, and future directions. Int J Med Inform. 2025;197:105838.
15. Burmann A, Fischer B, Brinkkötter N, Meister S. Managing directors' perspectives on digital maturity in German hospitals—a multi-point online-based survey study. Int J Environ Res Public Health. 2022;19(15):9709.
16. Wosny M, Strasser LM, Hastings J. Experience of health care professionals using digital tools in the hospital: qualitative systematic review. JMIR Hum Factors. 2023;10(1):e50357.
17. Pearson R, Beevers CG, Mignogna J, Benzer J, Pfeiffer PN, Post E, et al. The evaluation of a web-based intervention (Deprexis) to decrease depression and restore functioning in veterans: protocol for a randomized controlled trial. JMIR Res Protoc. 2024;13(1):e59119.
18. Stuart R, Fischer H, Leitzke AS, Becker D, Saheba N, Coleman KJ. The effectiveness of internet-based cognitive behavioral therapy for the treatment of depression in a large real-world primary care practice: a randomized trial. Perm J. 26(3):53–60.
19. Impact of the digital health application ViViRA on spinal mobility, physical function, quality of life and pain perception in spondyloarthritides patients: a randomized controlled trial | Arthritis Research & Therapy. [cited 2025 Oct 2]. Available from: https://arthritis-research.biomedcentral.com/articles/10.1186/s13075-024-03443-1.
20. LaBoone PA, Marques O. Overview of the future impact of wearables and artificial intelligence in healthcare workflows and technology. Int J Inf Manage Data Insights. 2024;4(2):100294.
21. Busnatu ȘS, Niculescu AG, Bolocan A, Andronic O, Pantea Stoian AM, Scafa-Udriște A, et al. A review of digital health and biotelemetry: modern approaches towards personalized medicine and remote health assessment. J Pers Med. 2022;12(10):1656.
22. Holmgren AJ, Esdar M, Hüsers J, Coutinho-Almeida J. Health information exchange: understanding the policy landscape and future of data interoperability. Yearb Med Inform. 2023;32:184–94.
23. Yeung AWK, Torkamani A, Butte AJ, Glicksberg BS, Schuller B, Rodriguez B, et al. The promise of digital healthcare technologies. Front Public Health. 2023;11:1196596.
24. Kreidler ML. The Development of Healthcare and Information Technology. 2023 [cited 2025 July 27]. The Development of Healthcare and Information Technology. Available from: https://www.ebsco.com/researchstarters/information-technology/development-healthcare-and-information-technology.
25. lee P, Abernethy A, Shaywitz D. Digital health COVID-19 impact assessment. 2020 [cited 2025 July 27]. Digital Health COVID-19 impact assessment: lessons learned and compelling needs – NAM. Available from: https://nam.edu/perspectives/digital-health-covid-19-impact-assessment-lessons-learned-and-compellingneeds/.
26. Ndayishimiye C, Lopes H, Middleton J. A systematic scoping review of digital health technologies during COVID-19: a new normal in primary health care delivery. Health Technol (Berl). 2023;13(2):273–84.
27. Abernethy A, Adams L, Barrett M, Bechtel C, Brennan P, Butte A, et al. The promise of digital health: then, now, and the future. NAM Perspect. 2022;2022 https://doi.org/10.31478/202206e.
28. Mansoor M, Ibrahim A. Telemedicine beyond the pandemic: innovations, challenges, and the future of digital healthcare. In 2025.

Importance and Impact of Digital Health Innovations

2

Jörg Traub

The trend toward individualization in medicine is increasingly shaping both diagnosis and therapy: instead of standardized approaches, personalized treatment strategies are coming to the forefront, tailored to genetic profiles, lifestyle factors, and individual disease progressions. However, this shift raises the critical question of affordability, as customized procedures and therapies initially incur higher development and application costs. At the same time, the move toward individualization significantly expands the pool of health data, which presents both a challenge and an opportunity. With the help of digital technologies and artificial intelligence, these large datasets can be analyzed and translated into clinical insights. AI-driven systems allow for the detection of patterns within complex data, making diagnoses more precise and therapies more efficient. Thus, digitalization is not only an enabler of individualized medicine but also a key prerequisite for making personalized care cost-efficient and accessible on a broad scale.

2.1 Most Promising Digital Health Technologies

Some of the most promising digital health technologies and application domains are artificial intelligence (AI) and Machine Learning (ML), digital therapeutics (DTx), remote patient monitoring and wearables, genomics and multi-omics platforms, as well as telemedicine and care platforms [1]. These technologies, supported by a robust evidence base, are rapidly transforming the realization of individualized medicine by harnessing digitalization for both clinical and cost efficiency.

J. Traub (✉)
HTGF – High-Tech Gründerfonds, Bonn, Germany

S. Scholz et al. (eds.), *Advancements in Digital Health and Care*,
https://doi.org/10.1007/978-3-032-16837-5_2

2.1.1 Artificial Intelligence (AI) and Machine Learning (ML)

These technologies power pattern recognition in huge medical datasets, enabling highly individualized diagnostics, risk prediction, and therapy optimization. AI-empowered systems are revolutionizing everything from genomics analysis to diagnostic imaging and clinical decision support, fostering both efficiency and precision in care delivery [2, 3].

2.1.2 Digital Therapeutics (DTx)

DTx refers to evidence-based software delivering interventions for prevention, management, or treatment of medical conditions. These solutions—validated through rigorous clinical trials—offer cost-effective, scalable, remotely delivered therapy (e.g., for diabetes, cognitive disorders, mental health) and can reduce disparities in access to personalized care [4, 5].

2.1.3 Remote Patient Monitoring and Wearables

Connected devices continuously collect individualized physiological, behavioral, and environmental data, enabling early detection, personalized intervention, and preventive measures. The resulting data pool enhances predictive modeling and real-time personalization, crucial for managing chronic diseases and fostering proactive, individualized care [6, 7].

2.1.4 Genomics and Multi-omics Platforms

High-throughput sequencing and omics integration platforms enable analysis of patients' genetic, proteomic, and metabolomic profiles. This underpins individualized risk stratification, early diagnosis, tailored drug selection, and monitoring of disease at the molecular level, thus paving the way for true precision medicine [8].

2.1.5 Telemedicine and Virtual Care Platforms

Telemedicine breaks down geographical and logistical barriers, facilitates continuous, individualized management, and enables timely specialist access. Integration of AI into telehealth platforms enhances personalization of medical advice and maintains continuity of care for patients with complex or chronic needs.

2.2 Shift from Diagnostics and Therapy Towards Prevention

Solutions in digital health and health data are shifting the focus from diagnostics and therapy toward prevention. Digital tools such as mobile health apps, telemedical monitoring, and electronic patient records are increasingly leveraged not just to manage existing diseases, but to proactively reduce risk factors for chronic illnesses. This paradigm shift arises from the recognition that preventative approaches, supported by digital technologies, can yield significant benefits for both healthcare outcomes and economic sustainability. For instance, in Germany, legislation such as the Digital Healthcare Act (DVG) allows for the prescription and reimbursement of digital health applications (DiGAs), which empower patients to monitor vital signs, manage lifestyle risk factors, and access preventive guidance before disease develops, yet only after confirmed disease upon prescription. The uptake of preventive digital health tools is further bolstered by the electronic patient record (ePA) rollout. This has the potential to foster a data-driven approach to population health and research.

On the EU level with the European Health Data Space (EHDS) and the regulation of the interchange of health data, digitalization efforts are reflected in programs that promote cross-border health data sharing. Besides primary use of health data, this will allow easier use of anonymized patient data for preventive research. However, the transformation is challenged by underinvestment in prevention: despite clear evidence that modifiable behaviors influence most health outcomes, only a small fraction of healthcare budgets is devoted to prevention. For example, only around 3% of OECD healthcare budgets are allocated to preventive interventions, highlighting the need for policy prioritization.

A concrete example of Germany's prevention-focused digitalization is the first reimbursement pathway for apps targeting early intervention in conditions such as obesity or diabetes. It covers, for instance, apps that guide users through risk self-assessments and behavioral modification programs. These apps, now accessible to millions through statutory health insurance via Digital Health Applications (DiGA), exemplify how digital health empowers both individuals and providers to shift from reactive treatment toward proactive health preservation [9–11].

2.3 Digital Health Provides Improved Accessibility of Healthcare

Digital health technologies, especially telemedicine and wearable sensors, have the potential to transform healthcare accessibility for rural and vulnerable populations by overcoming geographic, economic, and workforce barriers that have traditionally limited care. Telemedicine delivers virtual access to a broad spectrum of medical services, from primary consultations to specialist care, directly into patients' homes or community health centers in remote regions. Artificial intelligence (AI) can further support the early diagnosis and personalized communication and consultation. This innovation is crucial for populations where health facilities are sparse, distance to care is significant, and shortages in healthcare professionals are acute. Recent studies show that telemedicine increases patient satisfaction, reduces travel and associated costs, and facilitates earlier intervention for chronic and acute diseases, narrowing longstanding health disparities between rural and urban areas [12, 13].

Despite its promise, the practical integration of telemedicine and AI faces challenges, including broadband infrastructure deficits, digital literacy gaps, and regulatory barriers. To address these, many regions have invested in mobile health units equipped with telemedicine technologies, offering essential diagnostics and consultations directly to underserved communities. Case studies show that, in areas with robust telemedicine support, rates of timely specialist consultations and effective chronic disease management improve significantly. For example, programs providing teleneurology services in rural hospitals have dramatically reduced unnecessary patient transfers and improved care for conditions like stroke, where rapid intervention determines patient outcomes [14].

Continued progress requires focused efforts to close the digital divide and ensure telehealth solutions remain inclusive, especially for older adults and those with limited digital access. Policymakers and healthcare providers are now prioritizing investment in digital infrastructure and standardizing regulatory frameworks, aiming for universal, equitable healthcare access for all communities through digital health innovation.

2.4 Increased Efficiency and Cost-Effectiveness in Health Service Delivery

Digital health interventions, including independently usable health apps and telemedicine platforms, have been shown to enhance the efficiency and cost-effectiveness of health service delivery through streamlined workflows, reduced administrative overhead, and improved allocation of medical resources. Health economic evaluations increasingly demonstrate that digital health apps offer favorable cost-utility profiles, with several studies concluding these solutions are cost-effective compared to standard care, due in part to reductions in unnecessary face-to-face visits and optimized chronic disease monitoring. Systematic comparisons further reveal that, despite ongoing challenges regarding long-term evidence and standardized reporting frameworks, digital health innovations frequently lead to lower incremental costs per quality-adjusted life year versus conventional interventions, indicating significant potential for budgetary savings and for healthcare systems [15, 16].

2.5 Empowerment of Patients Through Self-Management Through Apps

Self-management apps are transforming healthcare by empowering patients to become active participants in their own health, fostering greater autonomy and improved outcomes. These digital tools enable users to monitor chronic conditions, track symptoms and medication adherence, and receive evidence-based behavioral guidance in real time. By offering personalized feedback and facilitating communication with healthcare providers, such apps strengthen patient engagement, support shared decision-making, and boost self-efficacy, leading to better health literacy and sustained behavior change [17].

One example of a DiGA that empowers patients is the HelloBetter program, which delivers digital cognitive-behavioral therapy (CBT) for patients with mental health conditions like vaginismus and dyspareunia. This app guides users through structured, clinically validated intervention modules, complemented by direct remote access to expert support. The program's evidence-based approach empowers patients to manage symptoms and improve mental well-being outside of traditional clinical settings, contributing to significantly enhanced therapy adherence and self-management capabilities [18].

2.6 Digital Health Solutions Driving Workflow Optimization and Interprofessional Collaboration

Besides direct impact on patients through, e.g., telemedical solutions, apps and wearables, there are also enormous potentials in workflow optimization and processes through digital tools.

These tools streamline administrative and clinical processes through automation and advanced analytics, reducing the burden of routine tasks on healthcare professionals and allowing more focus on patient care. Integration with electronic health records (EHRs) facilitates seamless information sharing among multidisciplinary teams, thereby enhancing communication and coordination across care pathways. A recent comprehensive review highlights that effective digital health implementations reduce clinician burnout by optimizing workflows, improving resource allocation, and supporting real-time clinical decision-making. Moreover, these solutions foster collaborative care models by connecting primary, specialty, and allied health providers through interoperable platforms, thus improving patient outcomes and operational efficiency [19]. The growing adoption of AI-enabled tools to automate scheduling, diagnostic support, and patient monitoring further enhances workflow efficiency and supports collaborative care environments, underscoring the transformative impact of digital innovations in modern healthcare systems.

2.7 Relevance for Public Health Surveillance and Chronic Disease Management

From a global perspective, digital health solutions have become increasingly important for public health surveillance and chronic disease management by enabling continuous, real-time data collection and enhanced patient monitoring outside traditional clinical settings. These technologies allow healthcare providers to detect disease exacerbations early, intervene proactively, and tailor treatment plans to individual patient needs, improving outcomes while reducing costs and hospital admissions. Examples are, e.g., health coach systems, which use AI-powered features including meal planning, sleep tracking, and medication reminders to support patients with chronic conditions such as diabetes and cardiovascular disease. These systems have the potential to continuously collect physiological data via wearable devices and integrate it with environmental factors to provide personalized care recommendations and predictive insights that anticipate disease progression. Such digital tools exemplify how the fusion of medical engineering and artificial intelligence can transform chronic disease pathways from reactive to precision, data-driven management [20]. Moreover, systematic reviews highlight the effectiveness of digital interventions for chronic diseases, showing improvements in self-care adherence and timely clinical responses that contribute to better public health surveillance [21], and telehealth platforms have expanded access to specialist consultations and remote monitoring, critically supporting population health and reducing disparities [22].

Digital health has already great potential in personal health, workflow, and process as well as public health. Yet its full power of big data, data fusion, and AI need to be implemented in everyone's life to improve health from therapy to prevention and from one-size-fits-all to personalized approaches.

Disclaimer The manuscript was prepared with the assistance of *Perplexity AI, Inc., Perplexity AI, Modell Sonar Large, 2025*, generative AI. Every section was carefully reviewed, revised, and approved by the author(s) to ensure that the text is appropriate concerning content and scientific correctness and maintain the integrity of the original content.

References

1. Berthold J, Hussain N, Zimic S. Top healthcare technology trends 2025. Avenga. 2025 Jun 17; Available from: https://www.avenga.com/magazine/top-healthcare-technology-trends.
2. Wang H, Li F, Liu Y, Guo P. Artificial intelligence and machine learning in precision medicine: a paradigm shift in big data analysis. Semin Cancer Biol. 2022;81:18–29.
3. Temple A, Lewis E, Hunt M, Redhead J, Kuang X. AI-powered precision medicine: utilizing genetic risk factor optimization to revolutionize healthcare. NAR Genom Bioinform. 2025;7(2)
4. Lin M, Ni C, Wang S, Yang H, Li B, Liu Y, et al. Digital therapeutics in China: comprehensive review. J Med Internet Res. 2025;27(1)
5. Murad M, Adler-Milstein J, Kumar S, Mohta NS. Review: characterisation of digital therapeutic clinical trials. Digit Health. 2024;
6. Piwek L, Ellis DA, Andrews S, Joinson A. The Rise of Consumer Health Wearables: Promises and Barriers. PLoS Med. 2016;13(2)
7. Lodewyk K, Hicks A, Noland K, Stratton SB, Kates E, Livesley N, et al. Wearables research for continuous monitoring of patient health outcomes in non-hospital settings: a scoping review. PLoS Digit Health. 2025;4(5)

8. Alsaedi S, Ogasawara M, Alarawi M, Gao X, Gojobori T. AI-powered precision medicine: utilizing genetic risk factor optimization to revolutionize healthcare. NAR Genomics Bioinf. 2025;7(2)
9. McKinsey & Company. Future-proofing German healthcare: Three catalysts to accelerate transformation. 2025. Available from: https://www.mckinsey.de/publikationen/2025-04-02-future-proofing-german-healthcare.
10. Germany Trade & Invest. The Digital Health Market in Germany. 2025. Available from: https://www.gtai.de/en/invest/industries/healthcare-market-germany/digital-health.
11. Goeldner M, et al. Digital health applications (DiGAs) on a fast track. J Med Internet Res. 2024;26(8):e59013. https://doi.org/10.2196/59013.
12. Anawade PA, Sharma D, Gahane S. A comprehensive review on exploring the impact of telemedicine on healthcare accessibility. Cureus. 2024;16(3)
13. Ashwini LH, Vinaykumar LH, Hanumanaik L. Telemedicine and rural healthcare access: a comparative analysis of emerging technologies. J Popul Ther Clin Pharmacol. 2024;31(11):169–79.
14. Zachrison KS, Richard JV, Mehrotra A. Paying for telemedicine in smaller rural hospitals: extending the technology to those who benefit most. JAMA Health Forum. 2021;2(8):e211570. https://doi.org/10.1001/jamahealthforum.2021.1570.
15. Kwasnicka D, et al. An overview on methods, evidence, and study quality of health economic evaluations of independently usable digital health applications. J Med Internet Res. 2025;27(8):e68349. https://doi.org/10.2196/68349.
16. Duffy S, et al. Comparison of cost-effectiveness between digital health interventions and conventional pharmacotherapy: a systematic review. J Med Internet Res. 2025;27(9):e70248. https://doi.org/10.2196/70248.
17. Bertelsmann Stiftung. Health apps. 2022. Available from: https://www.bertelsmann-stiftung.de/fileadmin/files/BSt/Publikationen/GrauePublikationen/SpotGes_Health_apps_en_final.pdf.
18. Madanian S, et al. Patients' perspectives on digital health tools: empowerment, self-management, and personalisation. Sci Direct. 2023;6:100051. https://doi.org/10.1016/j.hjdsi.2023.100051.
19. Loo RTJ, et al. Recommendations for successful development and implementation of digital health technology tools: a systematic review. J Med Internet Res. 2025;27(1):e56747. https://doi.org/10.2196/56747.
20. Dong C, et al. Precision management in chronic disease: an AI-enabled health coach system. Nat Rev Digit Med. 2025;2:30–42. https://doi.org/10.1038/s41746-025-01722-y.
21. Ambrosi E, et al. Effectiveness of digital health interventions for chronic disease management: a systematic review. EBioMedicine. 2025;78:103892. https://doi.org/10.1016/j.ebiom.2024.103892.
22. Centers for Disease Control and Prevention. Telehealth Interventions to Improve Chronic Disease Outcomes. 2025. Available from: https://www.cdc.gov/cardiovascular-resources/php/data-research/telehealth.html.

3 Overview of Key Challenges and Opportunities

Stefanie Scholz

The rapid evolution of digital health technologies offers unprecedented possibilities for transforming care delivery, improving patient outcomes, and making healthcare systems more resilient. Tools such as telemedicine platforms, wearable devices, mobile health (mHealth) applications, and AI-assisted diagnostics are reshaping how care is accessed, delivered, and evaluated.

However, these developments also bring significant complexity. Integration into real-world practice is hindered by structural, technical, socio-cultural, and regulatory factors that must be addressed for innovation to deliver sustained value.

This section provides a high-level overview of the most pressing challenges and most promising opportunities in digital health. It also sets the stage for deeper exploration in later chapters, where regulatory requirements (Chaps. 5 and 6), adoption strategies (Chaps. 8 and 9), AI-enabled transformation (Chap. 10), patient-centric reimbursement (Chap. 11), equity considerations (Chaps. 13 and 14), and emerging development paradigms (Chaps. 15 and 16) are examined in detail.

Understanding this landscape at the outset is critical, because—as later chapters will show—many challenges are deeply interlinked with the opportunities they accompany.

3.1 The Digital Divide: Unequal Access and Participation

Despite growing availability of digital health tools, access remains uneven. The "digital divide" describes disparities in the ability of individuals and communities to access, use, and benefit from technology [1–3]. Barriers may stem from:

S. Scholz (✉)
Faculty of Engineering, Ansbach University of Applied Sciences, Ansbach, Bayern, Germany
e-mail: stefanie.scholz@hs-ansbach.de

S. Scholz et al. (eds.), *Advancements in Digital Health and Care*,
https://doi.org/10.1007/978-3-032-16837-5_3

- Limitations in infrastructure, e.g., lack of reliable broadband in rural or low-income areas [4, 5]
- Economic constraints like inability to afford smartphones, tablets, or connected devices [6]
- Differences in digital literacy [1, 7]

Older adults often face usability issues with app-based health monitoring, while people in underserved or remote communities may lack stable connectivity for video consultations [8, 9]. Socioeconomic disadvantage, lower education levels, disability, and language barriers can intersect, creating "digital health exclusion" for those already at risk of poorer health outcomes.

This issue is revisited in depth in Part VII (Chaps. 13 and 14), which examines strategies to promote equity and accessibility for vulnerable and underserved populations.

3.2 Data Privacy, Security, and Ownership

Digital health depends on the collection and processing of sensitive personal health data. Safeguarding privacy and ensuring security are therefore central to building and maintaining public trust. A breach of medical data can cause significant personal harm, erode confidence in digital solutions, and lead to legal and reputational consequences for providers and vendors like the WannaCry ransomware attack on the UK's NHS in 2017 [10, 11].

Frameworks such as the EU General Data Protection Regulation (GDPR) impose requirements for lawful processing, data minimization, and cross-border transfer [12, 13]. Yet regulatory approaches vary globally, creating compliance complexity for solutions operating across jurisdictions (see Chap. 5).

Closely linked is the question of data ownership, whether health data ultimately belongs to the patient, the provider, or the technology vendor [14]. This debate has implications for interoperability, innovation, and commercial use. The European Health Data Space (EHDS), explored in Chap. 7, aims to balance secure data sharing for care and research with individual rights and patient agency.

3.3 Interoperability and Integration

Healthcare data are often siloed in fragmented systems: electronic health records, imaging archives, laboratory systems, and patient-facing applications. Without interoperability, the seamless and meaningful exchange of data across these systems—the full potential of digital health—remains unrealized [15].

International standards such as HL7 FHIR ("Fast Healthcare Interoperability Resources") provide a technical foundation for interoperability, but adoption is uneven and often hindered by proprietary system designs that create vendor lock-in

[16–18]. Poor interoperability not only limits clinical insights and coordination but also increases costs, duplicates testing, and impedes the development of AI tools that rely on large and diverse datasets [15, 19, 20].

Later Chaps. 8, 9, and 10 explore strategies for overcoming these barriers, including scalable integration architectures and collaborative, cross-vendor approaches.

3.4 Resistance to Change and Cultural Barriers

Even with infrastructure in place, technology adoption may be slowed by human and organizational resistance. For instance, Borges Do Nascimento et al. [21] found that clinicians may fear increased workload, question the clinical validity of certain tools, or feel uncomfortable with unfamiliar workflows. Concerns about job displacement or loss of autonomy can also play a role [22, 23].

Implementation science shows that successful adoption requires addressing both technical and cultural dimensions of change [24, 25]. Effective strategies include clear communication of benefits, participatory design with end-users, and training programs tailored to specific roles and contexts [26]. As Part III discusses, embedding digital tools into existing daily workflows—rather than imposing them as separate, parallel processes—tends to improve uptake. This is equally relevant in long-term and home-based care settings, which are addressed in Chap. 12.

3.5 Reimbursement and Sustainability Challenges

Many promising digital health solutions remain pilot projects because reimbursement is uncertain and long-term sustainability has not been planned from the outset [27]. Without consistent payment models or clear funding pathways, even effective solutions may fail to scale or endure, contributing to a system characterised by recurring "pilotitis" [28–30].

Germany's Digital Health Applications (in German "Digitale Gesundheitsanwendungen," or DiGA) framework seeks to integrate certain app-based medical devices into statutory health insurance reimbursement (see Chap. 11). However, challenges persist—rigorous clinical evidence is required for approval, uptake depends on physician recommendation, and sustained patient engagement can be difficult to achieve [31, 32].

Sustainability also concerns the technical lifecycle: many digital solutions become obsolete within a few years, requiring ongoing investment in updates, security, and integration [33].

3.6 Opportunities: From AI to Value-Based Care

While the challenges are significant, the opportunities for healthcare transformation are equally compelling:

- AI can support diagnostics, risk prediction, and treatment planning. If implemented responsibly, AI may improve accuracy, efficiency, and personalization—clinical studies show measurable, real-world benefits when AI is implemented under tight clinical governance. For example, the MASAI study found that AI-supported reading was non-inferior to standard double reading while reducing radiologist workload by ~44%; interim results showed ~20% more cancers detected without increasing false positives. Follow-up analyses in 2024–2025 suggest up to ~29% more detections and continued safety as deployment scales [34]. However, algorithmic bias, lack of explainability, and evolving regulatory requirements require careful governance.
- Personalized medicine, enabled by integrating genomic, clinical, and lifestyle data, allows more targeted interventions that can improve outcomes and reduce unnecessary treatments, but it also introduces data integration complexity and additional costs [35, 36]. Arnone et al. [37] indicate that PGx-guided prescribing can improve outcomes in several areas (e.g., antidepressant response/remission)—see also Chenchula et al. and Smith et al. [38, 39].
- Real-time data analytics, powered by data from wearables and IoT devices, supports proactive care, early detection of deterioration, and more precise chronic disease management. (e.g., heart failure: [40–42], COPD: [43–45], hypertension: [46, 47].
- Value-based care approaches link reimbursement to patient outcomes rather than service volume. Digital solutions can track performance metrics and facilitate quality improvement programs, but require alignment between financial incentives, clinical practice, and outcome measurement frameworks [32, 48–51].

3.7 Motivational Aspects and Gamification

Sustained patient engagement is often the deciding factor in whether a digital health intervention succeeds. Gamification, using game-design elements such as challenges, progress tracking, or rewards, can make health behaviors more engaging. It has been applied in contexts ranging from medication adherence [52–54] to rehabilitation [55, 56].

While gamification can boost short-term adherence, its long-term impact is less certain. Approaches must be sensitive to user diversity—competitive elements or design styles that appeal to some groups may alienate others.

3.8 A Matrix of Benefits and Challenges

The relationship between opportunities and challenges is rarely one-directional—each benefit is often paired with a corresponding risk that must be actively managed. Table 3.1 provides a short overview summarizing some aspects from above.

Table 3.1 Overview of selected digital health opportunities and their associated challenges

Opportunities/benefits	Challenges/risks
AI-enabled diagnostics and decision support	Algorithmic bias, explainability concerns, regulatory hurdles
Personalized medicine and targeted interventions	Data integration complexity, cost of genomic analysis
Real-time monitoring and predictive analytics	Data privacy, device reliability, patient compliance
Improved care coordination via interoperability	Lack of standard adoption, vendor lock-in
Value-based care enablement	Reimbursement model misalignment, outcome measurement complexity
Increased patient engagement through gamification	Short-term novelty effect, cultural inappropriateness, variable motivation
Scalable digital platforms	Sustainability of business models, rapid technology obsolescence

3.9 Navigating the Path Ahead

Achieving effective and equitable digital health integration requires more than technological readiness—it demands alignment between policy, practice, and ethics. Progress will depend on:

- Coordinated policy frameworks that both safeguard the public and enable innovation (linked to Part II)
- Adoption strategies that integrate technology into organizational cultures and workflows (linked to Parts III and IV)
- Ethical vigilance to ensure equity, autonomy, and trust (linked to Chaps. 4, 13, and 14)

Digital health stands at a crucial moment. The tools now available can support safer, more effective, and more inclusive care. Yet without deliberate governance, inclusive design, and forward-looking business models, these same technologies could deepen inequities, fragment care, or erode trust.

The rest of this book unpacks these themes, showing how actors across regulation, service delivery, and innovation ecosystems can work together to transform challenges into enduring, system-wide opportunities.

References

1. Jongebloed H, Anderson K, Winter N, Nguyen L, Huggins CE, Savira F, et al. The digital divide in rural and regional communities: a survey on the use of digital health technology and implications for supporting technology use. BMC Res Notes. 2024;17(1):90.
2. Kaboré SS, Ngangue P, Soubeiga D, Barro A, Pilabré AH, Bationo N, et al. Barriers and facilitators for the sustainability of digital health interventions in low and middle-income countries: a systematic review. Front Digit Health. 2022;4:1014375.

3. Yao R, Zhang W, Evans R, Cao G, Rui T, Shen L. Inequities in health care services caused by the adoption of digital health technologies: scoping review. J Med Internet Res. 2022;24(3):e34144.
4. Cuadros DF, Moreno CM, Miller FD, Omori R, MacKinnon NJ. Assessing access to digital services in health care–underserved communities in the United States: a cross-sectional study. Mayo Clin Proc Digital Health. 2023;1(3):217–25.
5. Maita KC, Maniaci MJ, Haider CR, Avila FR, Torres-Guzman RA, Borna S, et al. The impact of digital health solutions on bridging the health care gap in rural areas: a scoping review. TPJ. 2024;28(3):130–43.
6. Husain L, Greenhalgh T. Examining intersectionality and barriers to the uptake of video consultations among older adults from disadvantaged backgrounds with limited English proficiency: qualitative narrative interview study. J Med Internet Res. 2025;27:e65690.
7. WHO. Digital health divide: only 1 in 2 countries in Europe and central Asia have policies to improve digital health literacy, leaving millions behind [Internet]. 2023 [cited 2025 Jul 19]. Available from: https://www.who.int/europe/news/item/05-09-2023-digital-health-divide%2D%2Donly-1-in-2-countries-in-europe-and-central-asia-have-policies-to-improve-digital-health-literacy%2D%2Dleaving-millions-behind.
8. Wildenbos GA, Jaspers MWM, Schijven MP, Dusseljee- Peute LW. Mobile health for older adult patients: using an aging barriers framework to classify usability problems. Int J Med Inform. 2019;124:68–77.
9. Ahmad NA, Mat Ludin AF, Shahar S, Mohd Noah SA, Mohd Tohit N. Willingness, perceived barriers and motivators in adopting mobile applications for health-related interventions among older adults: a scoping review. BMJ Open. 2022;12(3):e054561.
10. Conduah AK, Ofoe S, Siaw-Marfo D. Data privacy in healthcare: global challenges and solutions. Digit Health. 2025;11:20552076251343959.
11. NHS. NHS England business continuity management toolkit case study: WannaCry attack [Internet]. 2023 [cited 2025 Jul 19]. Available from: https://www.england.nhs.uk/long-read/case-study-wannacry-attack/.
12. Federal Ministry for Economic Affairs and Energy. Guidelines on the Protection of Health Data [Internet]. [cited 2025 Oct 8]. Available from: https://www.bundeswirtschaftsministerium.de/Redaktion/EN/Dossier/guidelines-on-the-protection-of-health-data.html.
13. WHO Regional Office for Europe. The protection of personal data in health information systems—principles and processes for public health [Internet]. 2021 [cited 2025 Oct 8]. Available from: https://iris.who.int/bitstream/handle/10665/341374/WHO-EURO-2021-1994-41749-57154-eng.pdf.
14. European Data Protection Board. Study on the secondary use of personal data in the context of scientific research [Internet]. 2025 [cited 2025 Oct 8]. Available from: https://www.edpb.europa.eu/system/files/2025-04/20250401_study_on_the_secondary_use_of_personal_data_in_the_context_of_scientific_research_23102020_en.pdf.
15. Torab-Miandoab A, Samad-Soltani T, Jodati A, Rezaei-Hachesu P. Interoperability of heterogeneous health information systems: a systematic literature review. BMC Med Inform Decis Mak. 2023;23(1):18.
16. Ayaz M, Pasha MF, Alzahrani MY, Budiarto R, Stiawan D. The fast health interoperability resources (FHIR) standard: systematic literature review of implementations, applications, challenges and opportunities. JMIR Med Inform. 2021;9(7):e21929.
17. Littel G. Global FHIR adoption statistics: a comprehensive overview [Internet]. Co-Desion. 2024 [cited 2025 Oct 8]. Available from: https://codesion.com/global-fhir-adoption-statistics-a-comprehensive-overview/.
18. Gazzarata R, Almeida J, Lindsköld L, Cangioli G, Gaeta E, Fico G, et al. HL7 fast healthcare interoperability resources (HL7 FHIR) in digital healthcare ecosystems for chronic disease management: scoping review. Int J Med Inform. 2024;189:105507.
19. Imenokhoeva M, Lleonart L, Piha T. Harnessing digital health: analysing economic impact in healthcare systems - digital health advisory group for Europe report from annual high-level

meeting [Internet]. HIMSS EMEA; 2024 [cited 2025 Oct 8]. Available from: https://oregon.himss.org/sites/hde/files/media/file/2024/09/11/dhage-report_2024_v3.pdf.
20. Szarfman A, Levine JG, Tonning JM, Weichold F, Bloom JC, Soreth JM, et al. Recommendations for achieving interoperable and shareable medical data in the USA. Commun Med. 2022;2(1):86.
21. Borges Do Nascimento IJ, Abdulazeem H, Vasanthan LT, Martinez EZ, Zucoloto ML, Østengaard L, et al. Barriers and facilitators to utilizing digital health technologies by healthcare professionals. NPJ Digit Med. 2023;6(1):161.
22. Hassan M, Kushniruk A, Borycki E. Barriers to and facilitators of artificial intelligence adoption in health care: scoping review. JMIR Hum Factors. 2024;11:e48633.
23. Yew SQ, Trivedi D, Adanan NIH, Chew BH. Facilitators and barriers to the implementation of digital health technologies in hospital settings in lower- and middle-income countries since the onset of the COVID-19 pandemic: scoping review. J Med Internet Res. 2025;27:e63482.
24. Alzghaibi H, Hutchings H. Exploring electronic health record systems implementation in primary health care centres in Saudi Arabia: pre-post implementation. Front Med. 2025;12:1502184.
25. Rau E, Tischendorf T, Mitzscherlich B. Implementation of the electronic health record in the German healthcare system: an assessment of the current status and future development perspectives considering the potentials of health data utilisation by representatives of different stakeholder groups. Front Health Serv. 2024;4:1370759.
26. Finnegan H, Mountford N. 25 years of electronic health record implementation processes: scoping review. J Med Internet Res. 2025;27:e60077.
27. WHO. WHO guideline: recommendations on digital interventions for health system strengthening [Internet]. Geneva: World Health Organization; 2019 [cited 2025 Aug 13]. Available from: https://iris.who.int/handle/10665/311941.
28. Egermark M, Blasiak A, Remus A, Sapanel Y, Ho D. Overcoming Pilotitis in digital medicine at the intersection of data, clinical evidence, and adoption. Adv Intell Syst. 2022;4(9):2200056.
29. Schlieter H, Marsch LA, Whitehouse D, Otto L, Londral AR, Teepe GW, et al. Scale-up of digital innovations in health care: expert commentary on enablers and barriers. J Med Internet Res. 2022;24(3):e24582.
30. Kelley LT, Fujioka J, Liang K, Cooper M, Jamieson T, Desveaux L. Barriers to creating scalable business models for digital health innovation in public systems: qualitative case study. JMIR Public Health Surveill. 2020;6(4):e20579.
31. Mäder M, Timpel P, Schönfelder T, Militzer-Horstmann C, Scheibe S, Heinrich R, et al. Evidence requirements of permanently listed digital health applications (DiGA) and their implementation in the German DiGA directory: an analysis. BMC Health Serv Res. 2023;23(1):369.
32. Sippli K, Deckert S, Schmitt J, Scheibe M. Healthcare effects and evidence robustness of reimbursable digital health applications in Germany: a systematic review. NPJ Digit Med. 2025;8(1):495.
33. Gilbert S, Pimenta A, Stratton-Powell A, Welzel C, Melvin T. Continuous improvement of digital health applications linked to real-world performance monitoring: safe moving targets? Mayo Clin Proc Digital Health. 2023;1(3):276–87.
34. Lång K, Josefsson V, Larsson AM, Larsson S, Högberg C, Sartor H, et al. Artificial intelligence-supported screen reading versus standard double reading in the mammography screening with artificial intelligence trial (MASAI): a clinical safety analysis of a randomised, controlled, non-inferiority, single-blinded, screening accuracy study. Lancet Oncol. 2023;24(8):936–44.
35. Gladstone BP, Beha J, Hakariya A, Missios P, Malek NP, Bitzer M. Systematic review and meta-analysis of molecular tumor board data on clinical effectiveness and evaluation gaps. NPJ Precis Oncol. 2025;9(1):96.
36. DaCosta Byfield S, Bapat B, Becker L, Reyes C, Chatzitheofilou I, Schroeder BE, et al. Biomarker testing approaches, treatment selection, and cost of care among adults with advanced cancer. JAMA Netw Open. 2025;8(7):e2519963.

37. Arnone D, Omar O, Arora T, Östlundh L, Ramaraj R, Javaid S, et al. Effectiveness of pharmacogenomic tests including CYP2D6 and CYP2C19 genomic variants for guiding the treatment of depressive disorders: systematic review and meta-analysis of randomised controlled trials. Neurosci Biobehav Rev. 2023;144:104965.
38. Chenchula S, Atal S, Uppugunduri CRS. A review of real-world evidence on preemptive pharmacogenomic testing for preventing adverse drug reactions: a reality for future health care. Pharmacogenomics J. 2024;24(2):9.
39. Smith DM, Douglas MP, Aquilante CL, Deverka PA, Devine B, Dunnenberger HM, et al. Progress in pharmacogenomics implementation in the United States: barrier erosion and remaining challenges. Clin Pharma and Therapeutics. 2025:cpt.3736.
40. Scholte NTB, Gürgöze MT, Aydin D, Theuns DAMJ, Manintveld OC, Ronner E, et al. Telemonitoring for heart failure: a meta-analysis. Eur Heart J. 2023;44(31):2911–26.
41. De Lathauwer ILJ, Nieuwenhuys WW, Hafkamp F, Regis M, Brouwers RWM, Funk M, et al. Remote patient monitoring in heart failure: a comprehensive meta-analysis of effective programme components for hospitalization and mortality reduction. Eur J Heart Fail. 2025:ejhf.3568.
42. Parente HA, Hornemann SB, Faria IMD, Salgado DR, Correia MG, Azevedo FSD. Non-invasive telemonitoring programs for patients with chronic heart failure: a systematic review and meta-analysis of randomized controlled trials. J Telemed Telecare. 2024:1357633X241299156.
43. Mishra V, Stuckler D, McNamara CL. Digital interventions to reduce hospitalization and hospital readmission for chronic obstructive pulmonary disease (COPD) patient: systematic review. BMC Digit Health. 2024;2(1):46.
44. Stergiopoulos GM, Elayadi AN, Chen ES, Galiatsatos P. The effect of telemedicine employing telemonitoring instruments on readmissions of patients with heart failure and/or COPD: a systematic review. Front Digit Health. 2024;6:1441334.
45. Köksal N, Durgun H. Impact of telecounselling, home monitoring and exercise on hospital readmissions and quality of life in chronic obstructive pulmonary disease: a randomized controlled trial. Int J Nurs Pract. 2025;31(3):e70021.
46. Mehta SJ, Volpp KG, Troxel AB, Teel J, Reitz CR, Purcell A, et al. Remote blood pressure monitoring with social support for patients with hypertension: a randomized clinical trial. JAMA Netw Open. 2024;7(6):e2413515.
47. Teng T q, Sun G x, Yu Z y, Liu Z s, Wang T, Wu Q, et al. Efficiency of remote monitoring and guidance in blood pressure management: a randomized controlled trial: the role of remote monitoring in improving hypertension management. BMC Med. 2025;23(1):459.
48. Douglas AO, Senkaiahliyan S, Bulstra CA, Mita C, Reddy CL, Atun R. Global adoption of value-based health care initiatives within health systems: a scoping review. JAMA Health Forum. 2025;6(5):e250746.
49. Jackman L, Kamran R. Transforming patient-reported outcome measurement with digital health technology. Eval Clin Pract. 2025;31(4):e70107.
50. Schmidt L, Pawlitzki M, Renard BY, Meuth SG, Masanneck L. The three-year evolution of Germany's digital therapeutics reimbursement program and its path forward. NPJ Digit Med. 2024;7(1):139.
51. Benning L, Teepe GW, Pooth JS, Hans FP. Performance-based reimbursement for digital therapeutics in Germany: a misconceptualized opportunity. Digital Health. 2024;10:20552076241281199.
52. Nishi SK, Kavanagh ME, Ramboanga K, Ayoub-Charette S, Modol S, Dias GM, et al. Effect of digital health applications with or without gamification on physical activity and cardiometabolic risk factors: a systematic review and meta-analysis of randomized controlled trials. EClinicalMedicine. 2024;76:102798.
53. Yu T, Parry M, Yu T, Xu L, Wu Y, Zeng T, et al. Effectiveness of mobile health–based gamification interventions for improving physical activity in individuals with cardiovascular diseases: systematic review and meta-analysis of randomized controlled trials. JMIR Serious Games. 2025;13:e64410.

54. Tran S, Smith L, Carter S. Understanding patient perspectives on the use of gamification and incentives in mHealth apps to improve medication adherence: qualitative study. JMIR Mhealth Uhealth. 2024;12:e50851.
55. Bosch-Barceló P, Masbernat-Almenara M, Martínez-Navarro O, Tersa-Miralles C, Pakarinen A, Fernández-Lago H. A gamified virtual environment intervention for gait rehabilitation in Parkinson's disease: co-creation and feasibility study. J NeuroEng Rehabil. 2024;21(1):107.
56. Jiang Y, Sun M, Nuerdawulieti B, Huang X, Hou Y, Nan J, et al. Effectiveness of remote gamification pulmonary rehabilitation intervention based on the health action process approach theory in older adults with chronic obstructive pulmonary disease: a pilot randomized controlled trial. Front Med. 2025;12:1576256.

An Ethical Compass for Digital Health

4

Elmar Nass

An ethical compass for the use of digital technology and artificial intelligence (AI) in healthcare must neither focus solely on increasing acceptance nor be limited to questions of data protection. Instead of sales-oriented acceptance, the focus must be on normatively based acceptability. In addition to the certainly important issues of privacy, among others, the consequences of the use of technology for human image, responsibility, and human coexistence must be addressed. An ethical compass that provides normative orientation in the dilemma is thus inevitably tied back to ideology. This is because different implications arise depending on the normative content of the image of man and sociality as the value basis of ethics. This ethical discussion should therefore take up a very broad space in which, on the basis of religious, philosophical, or other substantive premises, many paths are transparently traced from the value basis to the concrete decision-making aid. The basic ethical direction adopted here reduces complexity. The proposed compass is based on a liberal-humanist ethic that draws on the traditions of the Enlightenment and Christianity on which the social market economy is founded.

4.1 A Question of Reasoning

Various attempts have been made to provide ethical guidance for digital health: (1) Reference is made, for example, to Isaac Asimov, who laid down rules to protect against malicious robots. According to these rules, robots must neither harm humanity nor injure people. Provided the first conditions are met, they must obey human commands and want to preserve their own existence [1, p. 47]. Asimov rightly asks about the consequences for humanity and humans. But it is not clear what harms humanity and people. (2) In 2022, UNESCO calls for the respect of universal human

E. Nass (✉)
Cologne University of Catholic Theology, Cologne, Germany
e-mail: Elmar.Nass@khkt.de

S. Scholz et al. (eds.), *Advancements in Digital Health and Care*,
https://doi.org/10.1007/978-3-032-16837-5_4

rights, the promotion of freedom, peace, and equality, as well as the protection of the environment and cultural diversity to regulate the use of AI [3, p. 6]. If respect for universal human rights is demanded, however, it must be taken into account that China's understanding of this competes with the liberal Western understanding. China puts collective human rights before individual human rights and thus wants to fundamentally change the world order and international law [6]. (3) Karsten Weber [10] and others presented the Model for the Ethical Evaluation of Socio-Technical Arrangements (MEESTAR) in the AAL context. It offers seven primary values or principles as a template, but does not define them in more detail. However, only when these criteria are filled with ideological content can they provide orientation for normative judgment. (4) The ethical principles of Tom Beauchamp and John Childress [2], which are at home in medical ethics, are also used as an ethical compass for the use of technology in healthcare. Four criteria (justice, autonomy, beneficence, non-harm) are intended to guide decisions in dilemmas. The principles are so general that it is still difficult to apply them in practice to evaluate the use of digital technology. After all, what does "fair" or "beneficial" mean? This requires differentiated interpretations in a more precisely identified value base, but this is lacking. It also remains unclear how a conflict of principles should be judged. In addition, the principles lack a clear justification-theoretical foundation. (5) The same applies to the European Commission's AI ethics presented in 2019, which, following Beauchamp and Childress, now demanded autonomy, harm avoidance, and fairness as principles and added explainability as a criterion [1, pp. 37ff., 3, p. 6]. (6) In the meantime, there are proposals to program a supposedly evident ethical orientation into robots or similar as so-called "artificial morality" ("AM"). It is thought to be the result of syncretic deliberation and is intended to relieve humans of responsibility in a dilemma. It also lacks a coherent justification and semantics for its criteria. It also disables human moral competence [7].

It becomes clear that, in addition to the existing approaches, a well-founded compass is needed to provide orientation for responsible people in concrete dilemmas. The liberal-humanist perspective is proposed here.

4.2 A Question of Acceptability

The normatively motivated push for increased acceptance in the digital health context carries the risk of subtle manipulation by commercial lobbies (Funk 2023, pp. 13–15). An ethical compass, on the other hand, must deal with questions of legitimacy for the use of technical innovations in healthcare. This form of acceptance, enriched by the aspect of legitimacy, should be understood as acceptability. The criterion for the ethical evaluation of the use of technology is not only its legal legality, its technical feasibility, or its economic efficiency, but also its legitimacy. The relevant definition by Klaus Kornwachs [5] is helpful for the fundamental semantic sharpening of this criterion:

> Acceptability is the result of a judgment regarding an action, its consequences, a fact, a motivation, an intention—in other words, everything that can be the subject of a moral evaluation. Acceptable is what conforms to one's own principles, values, priorities and adopted norms to such an extent that a possible conflict appears negligible. Acceptance, on the other hand, is an empirically ascertainable behavior of persons or groups of persons who actually tolerate an attitude, an action, etc., i.e. do nothing about it or consent to it (e.g. through purchase).[1]

The content of acceptability and thus the result of an ethical technology assessment depends on the transparent value basis of the assessor. This is made up of the following:

- An image of humanity and the associated understanding of human dignity (resulting in an understanding of freedom and justice)
- An idea of human coexistence and communication
- Addressees and contents of human responsibility
- An ideological source to be made transparent
- An answer to the relationship between human usefulness and the use of technology derived from all of this

Only with the help of this value basis can other relevant values and principles (e.g., in the approach of Beauchamp and Childress) then be prioritized, and concrete ethical assessments of the use of digital technology (e.g., AI) can be made.

4.3 A Question of Dignity, Sociality, and Responsibility

The ethical compass developed here belongs to the field of machine ethics and must weigh up the consequences of technology according to normative criteria. The starting point is the question of human dignity. This leads to answers regarding a culture of coexistence and responsibility. The diversity of human images gives rise to different ideas of human dignity and thus competing perspectives on ethics. The compass is therefore always perspectival. The perspective chosen here excludes the rationalization of human beings, whether this is based on the necessities of reason (Kant) or on the image of God (Christian). The use of technology must not sacrifice individual people according to collective or utility calculations. Living together is to be understood in an irenic way (as in the social market economy model). What initially sounds abstract can now be put up for discussion as a perspective compass contour:

Human dignity: Doctors who blindly trust AI in diagnosis and treatment, for example, become henchmen of technology. They reduce their patients to a billable data set. But people are more than that. Even cyborgs with AI brains are not human beings. The underlying optimization logic of enhancement devalues

[1] Translation by EN.

both human performance and people with flaws [1, p. 110, 3, 9, p. 39]. It subjects worthiness to a calculation of usefulness.

Sociality: When real and virtual life become blurred in the use of humanoid technology, inhibitions about violence and the motivation for social virtues decrease. The transhumanist repression of finiteness, for example, reduces the appreciation of old and dying people. Humanized robotics in care can also give the impression of human-like reasoning and genuine feelings. This could replace heartless and soulless human relationships. Such robots could also be used as trusting spies. If humans become something like "friends" with anthropomorphic artifacts and this trust can be exploited [1, pp. 82–85]. All of this needs to be taken into account, especially when using AI for people with cognitive impairments. AI as a colleague or even a boss would dehumanize the corporate culture and turn people into puppets of technology. If honest encounters are replaced by programmed empathy or "love," this creates a culture of lies, ambush, mistrust, and coldness. Generative AI produces unfeeling empty words instead of genuine relationships. However, the "social" must not be delegated to AI because this is essentially part of the profession of good human care.

Responsibility: AI or other digital technology should not be the bearer of responsibility. This presupposes freedom, reason, and morality, which it does not possess. AI-generated decisions, forecasts, and diagnoses are subject to the risk of manipulated data. This makes them susceptible to fake news. "AM" is not a solution to this. It is merely a syncretic calculation game in which there are no feelings such as shame, guilt, compassion, empathy or love, and certainly no well-founded values [8, p. 160]. Their decisions are therefore not fully comprehensible.

As we can see, people should take advantage of the opportunities offered by digital health, but must not allow themselves to become enslaved by it. It must remain an instrument whose results are evaluated and used by responsible people [8, p. 205].

4.4 Answers for Orientation

Human responsibility should absolutely frame the inherent logic of self-referential digital technology. The assessments must take into account the key perspectives of those directly affected or patients, those responsible for them and their environment, and the consequences for evolving images of humanity and society. The ethical compass offers the following basic guidelines:

- Technology that deactivates human responsibility must be rejected because it restricts people's scope of responsibility. This also includes technologies that only feign health and prevent people from consciously coming to terms with their frailty and the finite nature of life and consciously preparing for their death.
- Manipulation of people that significantly changes their integrity and responsibility should not be permitted: Imagine a digital technology that effectively

'implants' a new brain into a person. The assumption of responsibility presupposes freedom, but self-determination is not the ultimate criterion of acceptability. Personality-altering artificial manipulations, which could expand the scope of options and intelligence, are unacceptable if they undermine the continuity of human personhood and thus ultimately responsibility.
- Technological paternalism is a risk that must be taken seriously. Diagnoses and therapies must not be carried out solely by self-controlling algorithms, neural networks or quanta, because such systems no longer focus on people as individuals and reduce them to numbers and columns of data. Technology can and should have a relieving effect, but in the end decisions—even if supported by technology—must be made by people. The use of technology must not take on a life of its own, because technology has no soul and does not recognize a soul in the patient. It therefore cannot assume responsibility.
- The use of care robots as an aid is fundamentally acceptable. However, humanoid forms should be avoided wherever possible because they simulate human contact, manipulate emotional life and relationships, and contribute socially to relativizing the elevated dignity of humans in contrast to such machines.
- The following is also required:
  - Rejection of an evidence utopia associated with AI-generated results.
  - Rejection of anthropomorphic AI. To this end, it is helpful to use mindful language that avoids humanized attributions such as "learning," "autonomy," "experience," "social," "moral," etc.
  - Cultivating resilience against a dehumanizing logic of optimization.
  - Criteria for distinguishing between helpful assistance and harmful substitution of human relationships.
  - Ensuring connectivity between digital health and pastoral care with sick people.

In addition to this compass, researchers and users with a corresponding ethos are needed. "The focus must not be on the passive absorption of prefabricated material, but on the active mastery of complex judgments and decisions" [8, p. 161]. This requires intensive virtue training on dignity, freedom, and responsibility [4]. We need a broad ethical education initiative at schools and universities, especially in the so-called STEM subjects. Cultural differences must be taken into account here, such as animistic ideas in Japan, which attribute a soul to technical artifacts. Regimes such as China, which are driving forward a digitally supported synchronization of people, should also be be part of this discussion. However, anyone who refuses to comply with moral and legal standards must ultimately be sanctioned and ostracized.

References

1. Bartneck C, Lütge C, Wagner A, Welsh S. Ethik in KI und Robotik. München: Hanser; 2019.
2. Beauchamp TL, Childress JF. Principles of biomedical ethics. 5th ed. New York: Oxford University Press; 2001.

3. Funk M. Ethik künstlicher Intelligenz. Eine Topographie zur praktischen Orientierung. Wiesbaden: Springer; 2023.
4. Havens JC. Heartificial intelligence. Embracing our humanity to maximize machines. New York: Tarcher; 2016.
5. Kornwachs K. Philosophie der Technik. Eine Einführung. München: C.H. Beck; 2013.
6. Nass E. Der globale Puppenspieler. Die Vision von Xi Jinpinng und eine Antwort der Freiheit. Stuttgart: Kohlhammer; 2024.
7. Nass E, Schneider M. Maschinen mit Moral für eine gute Pflege der Zukunft? In: Pfannstiel MA, editor. Künstliche Intelligenz im Gesundheitswesen. Entwicklungen, Beispiele und Perspektiven. Wiesbaden: Springer; 2022. p. 311–23.
8. Nida-Rümelin J, Weidenfeld N. Digitaler Humanismus. Eine Ethik für das Zeitalter der Künstlichen Intelligenz. 4th ed. München: Piper; 2018.
9. Sandel MJ. What money can't buy. The moral limits of Markets. New York: Farrar, Straus and Giroux; 2013.
10. Weber K. MEESTAR2 – Ein erweitertes Modell zur ethischen Evaluierung soziotechnischer Arrangements. Conference Paper. Ostbayerische Technische Hochschule Regensburg; 2016. https://www.researchgate.net/publication/311699459_MEESTAR_-_Ein_erweitertes_Modell_zur_ethischen_Evaluierung_soziotechnischer_Arrangements. Accessed 6 June 2025.

Part II

Regulatory Landscape: Global Perspectives

5 Compliance Requirements for Digital Health Products

Christian Weigand

5.1 Introduction

The ongoing digitalization of healthcare is creating a new category of software-based medical devices that fulfil diagnostic, therapeutic, and preventive functions. Within the overarching term Digital Therapeutics (DTx), particular relevance is given to Software as a Medical Device (SaMD) and—specifically in Germany—to digital health applications (*"Digitale Gesundheits-anwendungen,"* "DiGA") and digital care applications (*"Digitale Pflegeanwendungen,"* "DiPA"). This chapter focuses exclusively on DiGA, as DiPA are subject to largely identical regulations but currently play a limited role due to less favorable reimbursement models. Compliance with regulatory and technical requirements is a prerequisite for market access, patient safety, and cost coverage in both the German and broader European healthcare landscape. The following sections outline the core regulations and detail specific requirements for DiGA—particularly those concerning data protection, security, and interoperability in accordance with the Digital Health Applications Regulation ("Digitale-Gesundheitsanwendungen-Verordnung," DiGAV) and the guidelines by the Federal Office for Information Security ("Bundesamt für Sicherheit in der Informationstechnik", BSI).

5.2 Regulatory Framework

The European legal foundation is provided by Regulation (EU) 2017/745 on medical devices (MDR) [2], which defines the conditions for placing software on the market as a medical device (Art. 2) and establishes essential safety and performance requirements (Annex I) along with procedures for conformity assessment (Annexes IX–XI).

C. Weigand (✉)
Fraunhofer Institute for Integrated Circuits IIS, Erlangen, Germany
e-mail: christian.weigand@iis.fraunhofer.de

S. Scholz et al. (eds.), *Advancements in Digital Health and Care*,
https://doi.org/10.1007/978-3-032-16837-5_5

In Germany, §§ 33a and 139e SGB V (Social Code Book Five, Statutory Health Insurance Act) [3] and the DiGAV [4] supplement the MDR with national reimbursement provisions. The Federal Institute for Drugs and Medical Devices ("Bundesinstitut für Arzneimittel und Medizinprodukte", BfArM) administers the so-called DiGA-directory and processes applications via the fast-track procedure. Depending on the device's risk class, designated Notified Bodies must be engaged for MDR certification prior to submission as DiGA. In some areas, for example data protection and data safety and security, the DiGAV goes beyond the requirements of the MDR. Therefore, these points should be considered from the outset when obtaining approval as a medical device or even during the development phase of a digital health application intended for DiGA registration.

5.3 MDR Requirements

According to MDR Annex VIII, Rule 11, software is generally classified as either risk class I or IIa. Conformity is demonstrated through technical documentation (Annexes II and III), encompassing development processes, architecture, risk analysis, and usability evaluation. Key standards include ISO 13485 (Quality Management Systems), ISO 14971 (Risk Management for Medical Devices), IEC 62304 (Software Life Cycle Processes), and IEC 62366-1 (Usability Engineering) [5].

Clinical evaluation (Art. 61 MDR) requires evidence of safety and performance derived from clinical data, which may originate from clinical studies, literature, or real-world evidence. Information security is considered a state-of-the-art, cross-cutting requirement integrated into the quality management system. Typically, these issues are addressed by implementing measures such as those formulated in the BSI's IT baseline protection catalog (IT-Grundschutz Katalog des BSI) [2].

5.4 Specific Requirements for DiGA

5.4.1 Status as Medical Device and MDR Conformity

A DiGA must be a medical device in a lower risk class (I or IIa), meeting the essential requirements of MDR Annex I. Therefore, at DiGA application at BfArM, the manufacturer must provide the EU Declaration of Conformity and, where applicable, a Notified Body certificate.

5.4.2 Integration with the Electronic Patient Record (*Elektronische Patientenakte*, ePA) and Health ID

The ePA is the central, patient-managed data repository within Germany's telematics infrastructure, enabling structured data exchange among patients, healthcare providers, and payers. Its interfaces and data models are specified by *gematik*.

Integration requires compliance with Medical Information Objects (MIO) [9] specifications which are based on the international HL7 FHIR standard. The MIO defines the structured transfer of medical data such as vaccination records, medication schedules, and laboratory results. MIOs consist of FHIR profiles, semantic terminologies (LOINC, SNOMED CT, ICD-10-GM), and validation rules. DiGA must fully support relevant MIO definitions (DiGA Toolkit) to write data into the ePA.

The MIO DiGA Toolkit provides a modular data model that can be used to transfer DiGA content (e.g., vital data, diary entries, questionnaires) from DiGA to the ePA.

In addition, the toolkit offers implementation and support mechanisms such as export examples, validation aids (e.g., HL7 validator), and formats for conformity tests and "connectathons" between systems.

The objective is to establish a binding and interoperable specification for the integration of DiGA applications into the ePA. This specification shall define standardized interfaces and processes while remaining implementation-agnostic, thereby allowing DiGA manufacturers sufficient technical flexibility. At the same time, it ensures uniform compliance and interoperability across all participating systems. The scope and content of the specification are intended to be subject to regular, legally mandated updates in order to reflect regulatory, technical, and functional developments.

Proof of write-access to the ePA and implementation of the Health ID is obtained via the gematik confirmation procedure pursuant to § 327 SGB V. Since May 1, 2024, this confirmation is a formal prerequisite for application completeness. Following directory listing, manufacturers must demonstrate activation of the SMC-B and registration with an Identity Provider (IDP) within 6 weeks [10].

5.4.3 Safety, Functionality, and Interoperability

The BfArM assesses whether an application is safe, functional, high quality, and interoperable under § 5 DiGAV. Safety and functional reliability must be documented through tests, error analyses, and evidence of stable software life cycle management.

Interoperability follows the cascade specified in § 6 DiGAV:

1. Primarily use KBV-defined MIOs.
2. If unavailable, apply open, internationally recognized standards (e.g., HL7 FHIR).
3. Publish proprietary profiles based on such standards in an open FHIR registry.

The MIO DiGA Toolkit must always be implemented in its latest version.

Where data from wearables or aggregators is used, interoperable interfaces (e.g., ISO/IEEE 11073, FHIR Personal Health Devices) must be provided to ensure device interchangeability and prevent vendor lock-in [13].

5.4.4 Data Protection and Information Security

To ensure especially data protection and information security, there are a lot of certificates standards and technical guidelines manufacturers must cope with. Here is a short overview.

Core requirements include:

1. Data protection certification since August 1, 2024, via a DAkkS-accredited body, based on testing criteria jointly defined by BfArM/BfDI [14].
2. Implementation of an Information Security Management System (ISMS) according to ISO/IEC 27001 or BSI IT-Grundschutz (200-2), with certification mandatory since April 1, 2022 [11, 12].
3. Mandatory penetration testing for all DiGA since February 1, 2024, preferably by BSI-certified entities, including white-box testing and manual code review, to be repeated regularly.
4. Use of cryptographic methods compliant with BSI TR-02102-1/-2, with selection justified based on protection needs and risk assessment [8].
5. In most cases, strong authentication (two-factor authentication, 2FA) in accordance with BSI TR-03107, providing insured persons with the digital identity pursuant to § 291(8) SGB V [7].

Compliance with BSI TR-03161 specifying minimum technical and organizational requirements for authentication, encryption, vulnerability management, logging, and security updates is also mandatory. Manufacturers of DiGAs and DiPAs must demonstrate compliance with data security requirements based on this technical guideline by January 1, 2025, at the latest, by submitting a corresponding certificate. DiGAs that are already listed but do not have a certificate will not be removed from the directory, but must submit this certificate as soon as possible. According to the new Guideline [1] v3.6 the ISO/IEC 27701 certification as an extension of ISO/IEC 27001 is now accepted as an interim standard.

Note At this point in time, there are unfortunately still no accredited certification bodies to carry out this certification in accordance with the data protection criteria. The processes for this are currently still in progress, and the submission of a certificate will only be required with sufficient advance notice once this is technically and organizationally possible. As soon as more specific time frames can be specified, these will be published on the BfArM website and the manufacturers of already listed DiGA will be individually requested to submit their certificates. However, it is recommended that you already familiarize yourself with the published data protection criteria of TR-03161 [6].

5.4.5 Proof of Positive Healthcare Effects (*Positiver Versorgungseffekt*, pVE)

Under § 8 DiGAV, proof of positive healthcare effects is compulsory for permanent listing in the DiGA directory. Typically provided via controlled clinical trials, pVE can be verified within 12 (extendable to 24) months after preliminary listing under the so-called fast-track procedure.

Since clinical trials must be well prepared, involve an ethics committee, and be monitored, manufacturers are advised to turn to an experienced digital CRO (clinical research organization). This CRO can conduct such a trial cost-effectively and, if possible, decentralize it, meaning it doesn't involve clinical centers. Decentralized clinical trials have shown significant cost-saving potential compared to conventional center-based studies.

According to a study by IQVIA, decentralized clinical trials can be conducted faster and at lower cost compared to traditional trial designs, with technology-enabled elements delivering measurable benefits for sponsors [16]. And the Fraunhofer IIS pointed out that digital decentralized clinical trials simplify participation by bringing the trial into patients' homes and enable broader recruitment and reduced dropout rates than traditional center-based studies [17].

5.5 Post-market Obligations

As MDR-classified medical devices, DiGA are subject to Post-Market Surveillance (MDR Art. 83–86) and vigilance requirements (MDR Art. 87). Software and algorithm modifications must undergo risk-based evaluation.

Changes to the DiGA that have a significant influence on the BfArM's assessment decision or that could lead to changes in the information in the directory are, in accordance with § 18 DiGAV, "significant changes" to the DiGA and must be reported to the BfArM.

The BfArM provides a checklist for significant changes for assessment purposes. If at least one of the questions listed there is answered with "Yes," it can be assumed that the change may be subject to reporting.

The checklist and the criteria listed in the guidelines are guidelines only—they do not release the manufacturer from its obligation to carry out its own assessment and, if necessary, consult with the BfArM.

5.6 Challenges and Outlook

The combination of MDR and DiGA-specific requirements increases development burdens for manufacturers but ensures a robust framework for safety, data protection, and evidence. Clinical study methodology for digital interventions remains a prominent challenge. Early planning and expert involvement are key to successfully demonstrating pVE, which is pivotal for listing and favorable positioning during price negotiations with the GKV.

Emerging frameworks such as the European Health Data Space (EHDS) and the EU AI Act present both hurdles and opportunities. AI in digital health applications is still in its infancy, facing stringent legal constraints due to the sensitive nature of health data. Nevertheless, anticipating EHDS technical specifications and integrating them early into product development may confer competitive advantage [15].

References

1. BfArM. Guide for Digital Health Applications –Version 3.5; 2025.
2. Regulation (EU) 2017/745 on Medical Devices (MDR).
3. Social Code Book Five (SGB V), §§ 33a, 139e.
4. Digital Health Applications Regulation (DiGAV), especially §§ 5–8.
5. ISO 13485:2016; ISO 14971:2019; IEC 62304:2006 + A1:2015; IEC 62366-1:2015.
6. BSI TR-03161. Security Requirements for DiGA (especially Chapter 4.2); 2023.
7. BSI TR-03107. Electronic Identities and Authentication; 2023.
8. BSI TR-02102-1/-2. Cryptographic Methods – Recommendations/Key Management; 2023.
9. KBV. MIO DiGA Toolkit and MIO Specifications; 2024. mio.kbv.de.
10. gematik. Confirmation Procedure according to § 327 SGB V and ePA Specifications; 2024.
11. BSI-Standard 200-2. IT Baseline Protection Methodology; 2022.
12. ISO/IEC 27001. Information security management systems – requirements; 2022.
13. ISO/IEEE 11073 Personal Health Device Communication Standards; 2021.
14. BfArM/BfDI. Certification Criteria according to Art. 42 GDPR (DiGA); 2023.
15. European Commission. AI Act; EHDS Regulation (Drafts); 2024.
16. IQVIA. (2022, September 7). New IQVIA Study Demonstrates Cost and Time Savings of Decentralized Trials. Retrieved from https://www.iqvia.com/newsroom/2022/09/new-iqvia-study-demonstrates-cost-and-time-savings-of-decentralized-trials
17. Fraunhofer IIS. (2025, February 5). Enhancing Medical Trials: Digital Decentralized Clinical Trials. https://websites.fraunhofer.de/smart-sensing-insights/decentralized-clinical-trials/

European Union Artifical Intelligence Act (EU AI ACT): Implications for Digital Health and Care

6

Elke-Luise Müller and Ute Irene Wiedemann

6.1 Introduction

The EU AI Act was published in the EU Official Journal on July 12, 2024, and entered into force on August 1, 2024. Since February 2, 2025, it has prohibited so-called unacceptable AI applications. The EU AI Act is legally binding for the member states of the European Union, while also setting global benchmarks [1]. As part of the European program for shaping the digital future of Europe [2] and a component of a broader AI package [3], which also includes an updated coordinated AI plan, the Act aims to provide AI providers, deployers, distributors, and operators with clear requirements for the use of artificial intelligence systems. Its goal is to harness the opportunities of AI while primarily safeguarding the fundamental rights of EU citizens.

Through a technology-neutral, risk-based approach, these objectives are to be achieved on the basis of the 2019 Ethical Guidelines for Trustworthy AI. Depending on the level of risk posed by an application to society and individuals, different regulatory requirements apply. Five risk levels are distinguished, each carrying different regulatory standards and obligations. Minimal-risk applications are subject to fewer obligations, while higher-risk applications are bound by stricter requirements such as transparency duties (e.g., AI-based chatbots, triage tools, or assistance systems). Certain particularly high-risk applications are considered unacceptable under Article 5 of the AI Act (e.g., social scoring).

In the healthcare sector, AI systems used in medical devices and health applications—such as diagnostic systems, robotics, and patient monitoring systems—generally pose potentially high risks to patient health, the protection of fundamental

E.-L. Müller · U. I. Wiedemann (✉)
DAK-Gesundheit, Hamburg, Germany
e-mail: elke-luise.mueller@dak.de; ute.wiedemann@dak.de

S. Scholz et al. (eds.), *Advancements in Digital Health and Care*,
https://doi.org/10.1007/978-3-032-16837-5_6

rights, and the secure processing of personal health and social data. Therefore, they require sophisticated risk analyses, effective risk management (Art. 9 AI Act), and conformity assessments, up to and including human oversight (Art. 8 ff. AI Act).

AI models with broad applicability, capable of performing a wide range of tasks and being integrated into numerous downstream systems, meet the criteria of so-called General Purpose AI (GPAI). Under Articles 51 ff. AI Act, GPAI systems are subject to additional, stricter requirements in cases of systemic risks [4, 5]. These provisions have been applicable since August 2, 2025. The regulations for high-risk systems will apply from August 2, 2026, while certain rules for products already governed by other harmonization acts will not apply until August 2, 2027.

Across all AI applications, the AI Act mandates that final decisions must always remain in human hands—automated decision-making without human involvement is explicitly prohibited.

6.2 Regulatory Compliance

Although the AI Act establishes an entirely new and unique legal framework, additional legal requirements at both the EU and national levels must also be considered to ensure lawful AI deployment that meets compliance standards. In contrast, legal systems in the Anglo-American sphere are based on common law traditions.

Since May 1, 2018, the EU General Data Protection Regulation (GDPR) has been in force, protecting and harmonizing the handling of personal data while strengthening data subject rights, particularly through increased transparency and ensuring a high level of data protection and information security [6]. Data subjects are granted rights of access and objection; data deletion policies and data protection impact assessments are required, along with the consideration of privacy in product and process design (Privacy by Design/Default). Furthermore, principles such as purpose limitation, data accuracy, and data minimization must be observed. Documentation and information duties complement the AI Act. Violations may result in fines, which can be imposed in parallel with penalties under the AI Act.

The healthcare sector is already highly regulated. In addition to the AI Act, the EU Regulation 2017/745 on medical devices (the Medical Device Regulation—MDR [6]) applies, along with industry-specific technical certification standards. To improve the use and availability of data for research and healthcare, Germany has also enacted the Gesundheitsdatennutzungsgesetz (Health Data Use Act—GDNG), effective since March 23, 2024, which enables the use of health data for public-interest research and the data-driven development of healthcare [7].

In the field of cybersecurity and information security, the EU Directive (2022/2555) NIS 2 [8] provides general standards of due diligence and liability for safeguarding networks and information systems. The AI Act complements these frameworks but also mandates harmonization. For example, manufacturers must demonstrate compliance with both MDR and AI Act requirements—particularly in the approval and market surveillance of AI-based medical devices.

Neither the GDPR nor the AI Act contains provisions tailored specifically to the healthcare sector and digital health services. From a compliance perspective, therefore, further legal development is advisable to optimize the legal infrastructure—also with respect to ethical concerns, ensuring the avoidance of gender-based, ethnic, or social discrimination [9]. This holds true regardless of the parallel goal of advancing data availability. Reducing legal gaps and ambiguities can not only strengthen technical safety but also lower barriers to AI use, improve quality of care, and enhance patient trust in the lawful and secure application of AI in healthcare, without hindering innovation.

The legal framework must also guarantee that, in the practical use of AI, final decisions are always made by humans, independently of the explicit requirement in the AI Act. In digital healthcare delivery, especially in the doctor-patient relationship, this is of paramount importance.

To determine the necessary and appropriate measures for optimization, user experiences, effectiveness, and the success of AI applications in digital healthcare must be measured in scientifically standardized ways, ensuring robust evaluation [10].

6.3 Description of the Different Risk Levels

The regulatory architecture of the EU Artificial Intelligence Act is visualized in Table 6.1. It is illustrated as a layered structure, with each line corresponding to distinct regulatory consequences.

The first level represents minimal-risk applications such as spam filters or entertainment-oriented technologies like video games. These systems are not subject to binding legal obligations beyond adherence to voluntary codes of conduct.

The second level concerns limited-risk systems, which include applications such as chatbots or recommendation algorithms. For these systems, regulation primarily focuses on transparency obligations—for example, the requirement to disclose that

Table 6.1 AI risk levels

Risk level	Description	Examples
Minimal risk	No binding obligation (only voluntary codes of conduct)	Spam filters, video games
Limited risk	Transparency obligation (disclosure, labeling)	Chatbots, AI-based recommender systems
High risk	Comprehensive obligations: Risk management Data quality Technical documentation Human oversight Post-market monitoring	Particularly relevant for healthcare Medical diagnostic software, AI-enabled medical devices, critical infrastructure
Unacceptable risk	Prohibited practices (with narrow exceptions)	Manipulative AI, social scoring by public authorities, real-time biometric identification in public spaces

Note: General purpose AI (GPAI) obligations (documentation, training date, safety testing) apply across risk level (limited, high and unacceptable)

users are interacting with an AI system. In healthcare-related contexts, subtle behavioral techniques (such as nudging in smoking cessation applications) may be permissible, provided that demonstrable health benefits can be shown and that individual freedom of choice is not unduly undermined.

The third level addresses high-risk systems, which are of particular relevance to healthcare. Within this category, the Act mandates comprehensive safeguards, including systematic risk management, requirements for data quality, detailed technical documentation, mechanisms for human oversight, and procedures for ongoing post-market surveillance. A pertinent example is software designed to analyze dermatological images for detecting potential malignancies. Because such systems directly influence diagnostic decisions, erroneous outputs may have serious consequences for patient health, thus justifying the heightened regulatory requirements. These obligations reflect the high stakes of medical decision-making and the potential impact of AI on patient safety.

The fourth level concerns unacceptable risk practices, which encompass applications deemed fundamentally incompatible with EU values. These include manipulative AI designed to exploit cognitive or behavioral vulnerabilities, systems for social scoring by public authorities, or real-time biometric identification of individuals in public spaces. Except for narrowly defined exceptions, such practices are strictly prohibited.

Finally, in addition to these four vertical categories, the Act introduces cross-cutting provisions for General Purpose AI (GPAI) systems, including large-scale foundation models such as GPT or LLaMA. Given their potential deployment across multiple domains and risk categories, such systems must comply with additional requirements regarding transparency, documentation of training data, and governance, since they can be integrated into all levels of risk.

This layered structure illustrates how the EU AI Act operationalizes risk differentiation: technical classifications are directly linked to legal obligations while being simultaneously embedded in broader ethical principles such as fairness, accountability, transparency, and patient autonomy. In the field of healthcare, this dual orientation seeks to enable innovation while safeguarding fundamental rights and public trust.

6.4 Technical and Medical Challenges, Opportunities, and Risks

Following the outline of the basic principles of compliance requirements under the EU AI Act, the focus now turns to the technical and medical dimensions. These aspects are not only of major importance for scientific debate but are also essential for the practical development, implementation, and regulation of AI systems in the medical context.

6.5 Technical Challenges

For high-risk AI, particularly demanding requirements exist regarding performance, robustness, explainability, non-discrimination, and safety. One of the central challenges is the control of algorithmic bias. Bias testing and continuous monitoring are mandatory to avoid discriminatory effects, for instance, with respect to gender, ethnicity, and socioeconomic background.

These requirements face significant technical limitations. Many machine-learning approaches, particularly deep learning models, are inherently characterized by the so-called *black-box problem*. Real-time monitoring and audits, as required by the EU AI Act, have so far only been partially addressed in research and demand new hybrid approaches in AI method development [12].

Generative AI models, increasingly used in both research and medical applications, require additional safeguards. Privacy-by-design mechanisms, differential privacy, and related safeguards must be further developed and consistently implemented in everyday medical practice to ensure that the handling of personal and sensitive patient data remains both legally compliant and ethically responsible [13].

6.6 Medical Risks and Opportunities

The potential of AI in medicine is considerable. Applications range from image-based diagnostics in radiology and pathology to predictive algorithms for therapy planning and digital health applications (DiGA). They can help refine diagnoses, individualize treatment decisions, and enable more efficient use of resources.

At the same time, the EU AI Act introduces additional regulatory burdens: high-risk AI systems are subject to external conformity assessments, documentation requirements, and continuous risk-benefit analyses, both prior to market entry and throughout ongoing use [14].

These obligations overlap with existing regulations such as the Medical Device Regulation (MDR), the General Data Protection Regulation (GDPR), and the Network and Information Security (NIS 2) Directive. As a result, manufacturers must demonstrate cumulative compliance with all requirements. This leads to significant cost and time burdens, particularly for small- and medium-sized enterprises (SMEs) and academic research institutions, potentially slowing down innovation dynamics [15].

Key Risks

- Overlaps and uncertainties between the AI Act, MDR, and GDPR
- Risk of slowing innovation due to high regulatory hurdles
- Cost-intensive conformity and certification processes, especially for SMEs and startups

Key Opportunities

- Strengthening of safe, ethically sound, and trustworthy AI applications
- Quality improvements through binding standards, external audits, and Conformité Européenne (CE) certification
- Building trust among medical staff and patients through enhanced patient safety
- Promotion of innovation via EU-wide "regulatory sandboxes" serving as testing environments
- Potential competitive advantage for European providers, as EU standards may serve as an international benchmark

6.7 Interoperability and Compatibility

A decisive success factor for the use of AI in healthcare is interoperability with existing information systems. The current landscape is highly heterogeneous: digital infrastructure and the start-up ecosystem differ significantly among the member states, and these are often driven by private initiatives [9]. To avoid missing interoperability and to support it at the EU level, joint platforms and projects are being promoted alongside legal and strategic frameworks.

Platforms such as MyHealth@EU serve as role models for a technical hub that enables the international exchange of patient data, e-prescriptions, and patient summaries among EU member states [11]. Compatibility with these platforms is therefore essential. For such initiatives to unfold their full effect, standardized technical formats (e.g., HL7, FHIR, SNOMED CT, ICD) and semantic standards (harmonized terminologies) are indispensable.

The obligation to ensure connectivity with these systems increases technical complexity but simultaneously creates opportunities for a more integrated and harmonized European healthcare system. Close cooperation among member states is crucial in this respect, in order to avoid inconsistencies in datasets and to ensure the long-term validity of AI systems.

6.8 Ethical and Societal Considerations

The European Union's Artificial Intelligence Act represents not only a regulatory framework for technical compliance but also a milestone in embedding ethical and societal reflection into digital health governance. Its provisions illustrate how the deployment of AI in healthcare is inseparably linked to questions of trust, fairness, autonomy, privacy, and social justice. In this respect, the regulation must be read as both a legal and an ethical document.

One central concern is the issue of trust and transparency. Healthcare professionals and patients alike must be able to understand, to a reasonable extent, how an AI system arrives at its recommendations or decisions. Without explainability, acceptance remains fragile, as "black-box" systems risk undermining clinical authority and patient confidence [15]. The EU AI Act therefore requires high-risk systems, such as AI-enabled medical devices, to be accompanied by clear documentation and mechanisms of human oversight, thereby operationalizing trust as a regulatory category [16]. This aligns with the ethical demand that technological innovation in medicine must be accountable to those whose lives it affects [18].

Closely connected is the problem of bias and fairness. Health datasets often reproduce structural inequalities related to gender, ethnicity, or socioeconomic status, which can translate into algorithmic discrimination [19]. In practice, such bias has already led to unequal treatment pathways and the reinforcement of health disparities. The AI Act addresses this by demanding rigorous data governance, documentation of representativeness, and continuous monitoring. Yet, as critics note, legislation alone cannot eliminate bias; rather, it must be complemented by active ethical governance and inclusive data practices [20].

Equally significant are concerns around autonomy and human oversight. The regulation emphasizes that AI is to support, not replace, professional judgment. This responds to the danger of automation bias, whereby clinicians defer too readily to algorithmic output. From an ethical standpoint, safeguarding human agency in clinical contexts reflects both the Hippocratic principle of "*do no harm*" and the need to preserve informed consent as a cornerstone of patient rights [18]. Thus, the EU AI Act embeds the notion that technological systems must remain instruments under human responsibility, not independent actors in medical decision-making.

Privacy and data protection constitute another critical field. AI in healthcare relies on highly sensitive patient information, raising concerns about surveillance, misuse, and erosion of informational self-determination. The Act reinforces the principles of the General Data Protection Regulation (GDPR) with AI-specific data governance duties, aiming to balance innovation and protection [18]. However, scholars argue that technical safeguards alone are insufficient; genuine ethical practice requires transparency in data use, accountability structures, and respect for patient autonomy beyond formal compliance [21].

Finally, issues of distributive justice and equitable access shape the societal dimension of the regulation. Complex conformity assessments and high compliance costs may privilege large corporations and well-resourced hospitals, while smaller providers and underserved regions risk exclusion. This could exacerbate the *digital divide* in healthcare, producing unequal access to innovation [20]. The Act therefore raises the broader ethical question of how AI can be deployed in ways that enhance, rather than undermine, solidarity within European health systems.

The EU AI Act addresses not only the technical classification of AI systems but also the distribution of ethical and regulatory responsibilities across different healthcare actors (see Table 6.2).

Medical staff are required to undergo training and ensure continuous monitoring of AI systems, with explicit duties for human oversight and incident reporting.

Manufacturers must implement robust quality management and risk assessment processes, supported by strict data governance, documentation, and cybersecurity obligations, alongside continuous post-market monitoring. Patients are granted transparency rights and protection of data sovereignty, ensuring informed decision-making and the ability to understand the involvement of AI in their care. In addition,

Table 6.2 Different actors face specific challenges when interacting with AI

Actors	Challenges	EU AI act requirements
Medical staff	Use of AI-based tools	Training, monitoring, control, incident reporting (Art. 73) Human oversight (Art. 14)
Manufacturer	Product development	Quality management, risk assessment, data governance, and documentation obligations (Art. 10–11)
	Technical	Robustness, accuracy, cyber-security (Art. 15)
Patient	Informed decision-making	Transparency rights, data sovereignty, right to explanation (Art. 13)
GPAI cross-cutting obligation Art. 54ff.	Post-market monitoring (Art. 72) for high-risk systems	Additional transparency and governance duties (Art. 53ff.), documentation of training data; risk and performance testing; support for downstream deployers in healthcare

the Act introduces cross-cutting requirements for general-purpose AI models, such as foundation models, demanding transparency, testing, and governance across all risk categories. Taken together, this framework connects the ethical concerns of accountability, fairness, and autonomy with concrete regulatory duties, ensuring that AI in healthcare is both innovative and socially trustworthy.

6.9 EU AI Act—Checklist

Implementing the EU AI Act in healthcare is not only a legal challenge but also an operational one. Hospitals, clinics, and manufacturers must translate abstract regulatory principles into concrete processes that can be applied in everyday practice. A structured checklist (Table 6.3) can help bridge this gap by turning complex requirements into actionable steps.

For practitioners, the value lies in being able to verify at a glance whether key elements such as data quality, interoperability, governance, and human oversight have been addressed. This prevents compliance gaps, supports patient safety, and ensures that innovation is not slowed down by uncertainty. The checklist also serves as a practical tool for project planning: it highlights where early investments in training, pilot projects, or transparent documentation will reduce risks later in the certification process.

By systematically working through these points, healthcare institutions and developers can not only ensure conformity with the EU AI Act but also strengthen clinical trust and accelerate the safe introduction of innovative AI solutions into real-world care.

Institutions must begin by clarifying their role as provider, deployer, distributor, or public authority, since these roles determine the applicable obligations [22]. High-risk systems, which include most AI-enabled medical devices, are subject to especially stringent requirements. A central element is the assurance of data quality and the adoption of recognized international standards such as HL7 FHIR, ICD, or

Table 6.3 Checklist for manufacturers and healthcare institutions

✓	Checklist item
☐	Ensure data quality and standardization: Adopt recognized medical standards (e.g., HL7 FHIR, ICD, SNOMED CT) and validate completeness and consistency
☐	Plan interoperability early: Verify compatibility with the European health data space (EHDS) and establish interfaces for cross-sectoral data exchange
☐	Establish governance and data protection: Define processes for access control, anonymization/pseudonymization, and audit trails; implement transparent governance structures
☐	Promote transparency and explainability: Document purpose, limitations, and system performance; provide understandable explanations to healthcare professionals
☐	Foster interdisciplinary collaboration: Involve clinicians, nurses, IT experts, legal and ethics professionals; jointly assess clinical, technical, and legal requirements
☐	Start with scalable pilot projects: Select use cases with clear, measurable benefits; ensure transferability and integration into larger systems
☐	Implement training and AI literacy: Provide continuous education for all professional groups; build a culture of trust where AI is seen as support, not replacement
☐	Anchor monitoring and evaluation: Define a post-market monitoring plan with clinical, technical, and ethical KPIs; regularly review outcomes and update processes

SNOMED, combined with systematic validation of completeness and consistency [16]. Interoperability with existing infrastructures, particularly with the forthcoming European Health Data Space, constitutes another essential pillar [20].

Governance structures are equally emphasized. This includes processes for access control, pseudonymization, and audit trails, together with clear allocation of responsibilities [19]. Transparency and explainability are identified as prerequisites for clinical trust: the purpose, limitations, and performance of AI systems must be documented in ways that can be understood by healthcare professionals [21]. In addition, human oversight remains indispensable. Physicians and nurses must receive adequate training and must always retain the ability to override or discontinue automated decisions, reflecting the ethical principle of safeguarding professional autonomy [16]. The Act therefore frames continuous education, often termed "*AI literacy*," as a legal requirement.

From an operational perspective, organizations are encouraged to begin with pilot projects that demonstrate measurable benefits while ensuring scalability and integration into larger clinical systems. Continuous post-market monitoring is mandated, assessing clinical, technical, and ethical dimensions, and serious incidents must be reported to authorities within strict timelines [20]. Moreover, procurement contracts with manufacturers should explicitly cover EU AI Act obligations, including documentation, support for conformity assessments, and guarantees of transparency.

Taken together, the EU AI Act connects legal compliance with broader ethical and societal principles. By enforcing standards for data quality, interoperability, transparency, human oversight, and monitoring, the Act seeks to reinforce trust and accountability while simultaneously enabling innovation. Healthcare institutions that align their practices with these requirements not only ensure conformity with EU law but also contribute to a more reliable and ethically grounded use of artificial intelligence in medicine [17, 20].

6.10 Conclusion

The EU AI Act marks a decisive turning point in the regulation of artificial intelligence. With its entry into force in 2024 and the staggered implementation of its provisions through 2027, it has created, for the first time, a coherent, EU-wide legal framework that not only formulates technical requirements but also integrates them with ethical guiding principles. Designed as a technology-neutral, risk-based approach, it represents an innovative response to the need to systematically harness the opportunities of AI while effectively protecting citizens' fundamental rights. The differentiation by risk levels—ranging from minimal to limited to high risk, along with the explicit prohibition of unacceptable practices—ensures that regulatory intervention is graduated according to the potential harms to individuals and society.

In healthcare, these provisions have particularly far-reaching effects. AI systems that support diagnosis, plan therapies, or monitor patients hold significant potential to improve quality of care and increase efficiency in resource use. At the same time, however, they carry risks for patient safety, data protection, and fundamental rights. Accordingly, they are subject to strict requirements regarding risk management, data quality, transparency, and human oversight. For general-purpose AI models, which are increasingly applied in medicine, additional heightened requirements apply, given their wide applicability and potential systemic risks.

The embedding of the AI Act within a network of existing European legal frameworks—including the GDPR, the Medical Device Regulation (MDR), the NIS 2 Directive, and the Health Data Use Act (GDNG)—demonstrates that it does not stand alone but rather functions as a complementary body of law. While this interconnection strengthens legal certainty, it also increases regulatory complexity. For manufacturers, healthcare providers, and research institutions, this entails substantial organizational and financial burdens. Smaller actors, such as startups and SMEs, in particular, may see their innovative capacity restricted by high costs and lengthy certification processes.

Despite these challenges, the Act offers significant opportunities. Obligations for transparency, documentation, and external oversight can strengthen trust among patients and healthcare professionals. Binding quality standards foster robustness and safety in systems and may position Europe as an international leader. The AI Act is therefore not only a tool for risk mitigation but also a potential driver of innovation: companies that invest in compliance may benefit from competitive advantages, especially if the European standard is adopted globally as a benchmark.

Beyond its regulatory function, the Act has a normative dimension. It clearly signals that AI applications in healthcare must remain instruments of human decision-making. The risk of *automation bias*—the uncritical adoption of algorithmic outputs by physicians—is addressed through the requirement of final human responsibility. Likewise, combating algorithmic bias and structural discrimination is an integral part of the regulation, underscoring the commitment to fair and inclusive AI deployment.

Interoperability remains of central importance. Only if AI systems can be seamlessly integrated with electronic health records, clinical information systems, and European data platforms such as MyHealth@EU or the emerging European Health Data Space will their full potential and scalability be realized. Standardized technical formats (HL7 FHIR, SNOMED CT, ICD) and semantic interoperability are indispensable in this respect.

Thus, the implementation of the EU AI Act does not represent an endpoint but the beginning of a new phase of development. Open challenges particularly concern the development of practical methods for explainable AI, the standardization of audits and conformity assessments, the design of human-machine interactions in clinical practice, and the scientifically sound evaluation of efficacy and safety. Mechanisms must also be established to ensure that the digital divide between large, financially strong providers and smaller institutions does not deepen, thereby safeguarding equitable access to innovation in healthcare.

Overall, the EU AI Act brings together technical innovation, regulatory accountability, and societal values into a comprehensive framework for digital healthcare. Its success will ultimately be measured by whether it can improve quality of care, protect patient safety and fundamental rights, and at the same time create an innovation-friendly environment. In doing so, the Act provides not only a legal foundation but also a normative orientation for the responsible, just, and sustainable use of AI in healthcare—and lays the groundwork for Europe's potential leadership role in the global development of medical AI systems.

References

1. https://eur-lex.europa.eu EU Law and related documents; open data from the EU The Open Data Portal (http://data.europa.eu/euodp/en) EU publications https://publications.europa.eu/en/publications
2. European Commission (2025), A Europe fit for the digital age, https://commission.europa.eu/strategy-and-policy/priorities-2019-2024/europe-fit-digital-age/shaping-europes-digital-future_de.
3. https://digital-strategy.ec.europa.eu/de/policies/european-approach-artificial-intelligence.
4. Ammann T, Pohle J (2024) Compliance-Berater, 137–142
5. Ammann T, Plote M, Schmechel P (2024), Compliance-Berater, 317–320
6. https://eur-lex.europa.eu.
7. https://www.bundesgesundheitsministerium.de.
8. https://digital-strategy.ec.europa.eu.
9. European Commission (2021) Study on eHealth, interoperability of health data and artificial intelligence for health and care in the European Union, Lot 2: artificial intelligence for health and care in the EU country factsheets. Luxembourg: Publications Office of the European Union
10. Hammer J, Flok A, Herberg S, Teuteberg F (2025) Navigating the complexity of evaluating artificial intelligence in healthcare, Ecis 2025 Proceedings 11. https://aisel.aisnet.org/cgi/viewcontent.cgi?article=1170&context=ecis2025

11. European Commission. Elektronische grenzüberschreitende Gesundheitsdienste(2025), https://health.ec.europa.eu/ehealth-digital-health-and-care/digital-health-and-care/electronic-cross-border-health-services_de
12. Schmid U (2024) Trustworthy artificial intelligence: comprehensible, transparent and correctable. In: Werthner H, et al., editors. Introduction to digital humanism. Cham: Springer; https://doi.org/10.1007/978-3-031-45304-5_10
13. European Commission: What does data protection "by design" and "by default" mean? https://commission.europa.eu/law/law-topic/data-protection/rules-business-and-organisations/obligations/what-does-data-protection-design-and-default-mean_en#examples
14. Medizinischer Dienst Bund (2025) Künstliche Intelligenz im Medizinprodukten: Neue Herausforderungen durch den „AI-Act" der EU, 2025-05-05_Kuenstliche_Intelligenz_in_Medizinprodukten.pdf.
15. Segschneider A (2024) EU Verordnung AI Act: Regulierung von KI im Gesundheitswesen. AI-Act: Regulierung von KI im Gesundheitswesen - Wegweiser Regulatorik Gesundheitswirtschaft BW
16. Mittelstadt, B (2019) Principles alone cannot guarantee ethical AI. Nature Machine Intelligence, 1(11), 501–507. https://doi.org/10.1038/s42256-019-0114-4
17. European Commission (2021) Ethics of Artificial Intelligence in Health Care. European Group on Ethics in Science and New Technologies.
18. Obermeyer Z, Powers B, Vogeli C, & Mullainathan S (2019) Dissecting racial bias in an algorithm used to manage the health of populations. Science, 366(6464), 447–453. https://doi.org/10.1126/science.aax2342
19. Vayena E, Blasimme A, & Cohen I G (2018) Machine learning in medicine: Addressing ethical challenges. PLoS Medicine, 15(11), e1002689. https://doi.org/10.1371/journal.pmed.1002689
20. European Group on Ethics in Science and New Technologies (2021) Opinion on the Ethics of Artificial Intelligence in Healthcare. European Commission.
21. Morley J, Machado CC, Burr C, Cowls J, Joshi I, Taddeo M, Floridi M (2020) The ethics of AI in health care: a mapping review. Soc Sci Med.;260:113172. https://doi.org/10.1016/j.socscimed.2020.113172

7 Health Data with the European Health Data Space (EHDS)

Kurt Höller and Lisa Walter

Why the introduction of the European Health Data Space (EHDS) was long overdue, what it includes and what it doesn't, the opportunities it now presents for society, healthcare providers, and the economy, and what must be considered during its implementation—an optimistic overall perspective [1].

Background—All European countries are united in shaping the legal framework for health data.

When the European Union's General Data Protection Regulation (GDPR) [2] came into force in 2018—referred to in Germany as the Datenschutzgrundverordnung (DSGVO)—lawmakers deliberately chose not to include specific provisions governing the use of medical data. The risk was simply too great that one of the European Member States, due to different views in this highly specific area, might have blocked the implementation of the entire GDPR with a veto. Yet, it is precisely the handling of medical information that demands special attention—not only to protect sensitive personal health data but also to unlock tremendous potential for innovation. This deliberate omission created a regulatory vacuum in secondary data use for research and innovation, which the EHDS now seeks to fill. If this health data can be used responsibly, across borders, and within clearly defined frameworks, it will improve healthcare delivery and advance research and development throughout Europe. Thus, it became increasingly important to launch a suitable cross-border legal framework for this domain.

K. Höller (✉)
Healthcare Vertical Market, Siemens AG, Erlangen, Germany

CiNNAMED GmbH, Erlangen, Germany
e-mail: kurt.hoeller@siemens.com

L. Walter
EIT Health Germany-Switzerland GmbH, Munich, Germany

S. Scholz et al. (eds.), *Advancements in Digital Health and Care*,
https://doi.org/10.1007/978-3-032-16837-5_7

7.1 The History of European Health Data Space

In December 2019, when appointing her Commissioners, EU President Ursula von der Leyen clearly outlined the cornerstones of a European Health Data Space in a mission letter to Commissioner Stella Kyriakides, in her role as Commissioner for Health and Food Safety [3]. "I want you to work on the creation of a European Health Data Space to promote health-data exchange and support research on new preventive strategies, as well as on treatments, medicines, medical devices and outcomes. As part of this, you should ensure citizens have control over their own personal data."

The geopolitical reasoning behind the EHDS is deeply embedded within the broader European Data Strategy, which was published by the European Commission in February 2020, shortly after President von der Leyen's mission letter. It explicitly outlines the EU's ambition to become a leader in the data economy and to assert its digital sovereignty and autonomy, reducing dependence on non-EU tech giants [4]. The EHDS is a critical component of this, ensuring sensitive health data remains under European control. The relevance of digital healthcare became evident during the COVID-19 pandemic, which accelerated adoption across Europe. Doctors' and patients' willingness to embrace digital solutions in parallel with the integration of digital tools into everyday life, from video conferencing to the COVID tracking app, reinforced their value.

With the entry into force of the Digital Healthcare Act (DVG) on December 19, 2019, Germany for example had already created the legal basis for the prescription and reimbursement of digital health applications (DiGAs) at an early stage and also set mandatory IT security standards. A wide range of "well-being" applications already existed, such as those for online meditation or virtual fitness coaching, which always must be paid for by the user themself. Now more startups are also setting out to reimburse new applications—certified as Class I or IIa medical devices. Once they pass an initial review and are approved by the Federal Institute for Drugs and Medical Devices (BfArM), they are listed as DiGAs. The startups then have 12 months to prove their effectiveness [5].

Even though Germany has made a real leap forward in innovation, one that even prompted President Emmanuel Macron not only to take the German DiGA system as a model but also to actively replicate it in France as so-called PECAN already since April 2023 [6], the German healthcare system still has a long road ahead.

The Commission's proposal marks an ambitious yet long-anticipated step toward harmonizing cross-border health data exchange. The legislative proposal which was published by the European Commission on May 3, 2022, the creation of a European Health Data Space [7] clearly demonstrated that this initiative, as a key building block for a sustainable and resilient European Health Union, holds the fundamental potential to significantly strengthen Europe's capacity for innovation in the field of digital health and to overcome existing barriers.

After extensive negotiations around the balance between EU and national governance (with European Council and European Parliament reinforcing national Health Data Access Bodies), and the scope and restrictions on commercial access to health data (with both Council and Parliament introducing stricter limitations than the Commission's initial proposal), the Council agreed to its position in December 2023, and by March 15, 2024, the European Parliament and the Council had reached a provisional agreement [8, 9]. This addressed key debates around access rights, interoperability, opt-outs, and data governance. The regulation was formally adopted as Regulation (EU) 2025/327, published in the Official Journal on March 5, 2025, and entered into force on March 26, 2025 [10]. This marked a decisive shift from discussion to implementation.

7.2 The European Exchange of Healthcare Data under Citizen Ownership and Control

At its core, the EHDS creates the much-needed framework for balancing patients' rights on the one hand and the needs of innovators on the other. From the patients' point of view, it is not only important to have control over their own data but also to finally be able to fully access it themselves and, for the purpose of their own treatment, to grant access to medical personnel ("primary use"). At the same time, however, this framework also takes into account the requirements of innovators and decision makers in the healthcare industry, science, research, and politics. By using aggregated healthcare data, they are now empowered to transform healthcare as a whole and thereby offer additional value to society (not only in the treatment of patients, but also in the prevention for healthy citizens) ("secondary use") (Fig. 7.1). The EHDS factsheet also explicitly highlights the economic significance of a single market for digital health services and products ("Unleash the data economy by fostering a genuine single market for digital health services and products") [11].

The Commission frequently employs illustrative scenarios to elucidate the patient-centric vision of its new framework. As detailed in an online publication [12], three examples articulate this perspective. Firstly, the framework enables a healthcare provider to access and comprehend a patient's structured medical history across linguistic and national borders, facilitating informed pharmacotherapy and

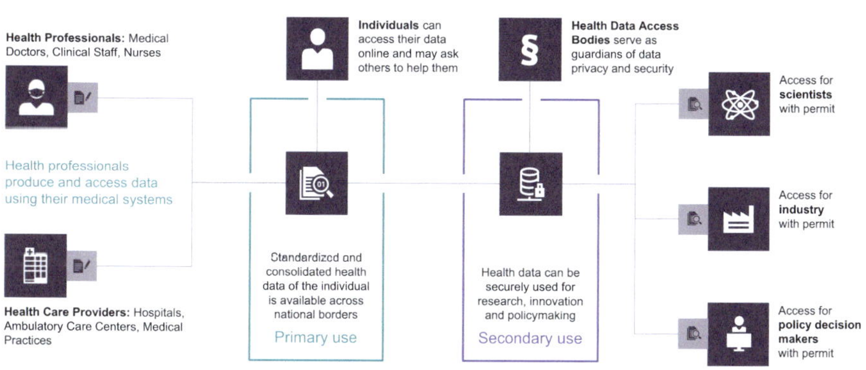

Fig. 7.1 Primary and secondary use of electronic health records in the context of the EHDS; (Source: Own illustration)

mitigating risks from intolerances or allergies. Secondly, it provides technology companies, within initiatives like the EHDS, secure and efficient access to extensive, anonymized datasets for training and validating artificial intelligence algorithms, thereby enhancing diagnostic and treatment efficacy. Thirdly, the framework empowers patients to authorize secure access to their own medical data, such as diagnostic imaging, across different healthcare institutions, preventing redundant procedures, minimizing radiation exposure, and optimizing healthcare resource utilization.

From the citizen's perspective, the EHDS enshrines the right to access personal electronic health data across the EU and to control its use. Opt-outs for secondary use are foreseen in some contexts. At the same time, strict safeguards exclude misuse, such as by insurers for premium calculations. In an EHDS background document of the Commission [13] it becomes clear that the Commission also recognizes the urgent need for citizens' trust in the system as a basic prerequisite for the success of the EHDS: "Trust as the foundation of the European Health Data Space." This is not only about legally anchored data protection but also about technologically anchored cybersecurity, which not only enables access by the patient in a fast, free and technically simple way but also records who else has accessed the health data and for what purpose. Transparency measures, including audit trails of data access, aim to build trust.

The EHDS itself does not provide a single technological solution, but defines the requirements, for example, for an electronic health record. This approach highlights Europe's commitment to federalized data models, where implementation remains the responsibility of the Member States themselves, thereby differing significantly from more centralized architectures. This strategy aligns with the core principles of initiatives like Gaia-X [14], which aims to establish a secure, federated, and interoperable data infrastructure across Europe, emphasizing data sovereignty and user control over centralized monolithic systems [15]. Electronic health record systems across Europe must comply with the European electronic health record exchange format, ensuring structured, multilingual, cross-border data use. In addition to the patient file, information from the medical care environment is also required, such as image data, electronic prescriptions, or telemedicine records. The integration of well-being and health applications on citizens' mobile phones is also being sought to obtain holistic disease patterns or prevention basics. All Member States will be obliged to participate in the cross-border digital infrastructure "MyHealth@EU," which is intended to ensure an effective exchange of patient data for the purpose of care (primary use). Germany's National Digital Health Agency, gematik, plays a crucial role in providing core telematics infrastructure services and contributing to the MyHealth@EU platform [16]. In addition, a new "European Health Data Space Board" led by the Commission with the involvement of all Digital Health Authorities in the Member States is to monitor the rule-compliant introduction. The EHDS Board has proposed the establishment of two Steering Groups to manage cross-border digital infrastructures (primary and secondary use).

The think tank report "Learning from health data use cases: Real-world challenges and enablers to the creation of the EHDS," published by EIT Health in 2021

[17], urges policymakers to consider the following three key elements for creating a truly functional EHDS: Effectively Mapping the Roles of Health Data Users, Data Interoperability Compliance and Monitoring, as well as Clear Legislation avoiding Overlaps and Over-Regulation to simplify Compliance. These demands remain valid and will be presented again below [18].

7.3 Effectively Mapping the Roles of Health Data Users

The EHDS Governance Framework must effectively consider the different roles of health data users, discuss them with all stakeholders, and reconcile them. Although the way in which health data is accessed and used is determined by the role of the user in the healthcare system, these roles are not static: medical staff can also conduct research; representatives of statutory health insurance companies can also be involved in political decision-making processes; and every citizen can also be a patient, a family caregiver, or even a donor of data. The EHDS Stakeholder Forum is an envisioned platform for gathering insights from citizens, healthcare professionals, patient organizations, researchers, and industry to foster trust and support the consistent application of the EHDS Regulation throughout the EU.

All of this requires a regulatory framework that enables a smooth transition of roles and responsibilities for all stakeholders, while consistently prioritizing the rights and interests of patients. This must be reflected both in the European framework and in its national implementation, including legislative processes in the German Bundestag. Broad acceptance and meaningful adoption can only be achieved through the active involvement of representatives from all relevant groups. The overarching goal would be fundamentally undermined if large segments of the population opted out of secondary use or if data access were so restricted that it no longer provided meaningful value for innovation.

7.4 Data Interoperability Compliance and Monitoring

Emphasis must be placed on data interoperability as a central pillar across different technologies and national borders. The practices and standards for the collection, processing, and storage of health data vary greatly depending on countries and areas, which naturally pose major challenges for interoperability, thus demanding a comprehensive strategy that distinguishes syntactic interoperability (the ability of systems to exchange and parse data, often via structured formats like HL7, FHIR, and ISO/IEEE 11073), semantic interoperability (ensuring the consistent understanding of data's meaning, exemplified by SNOMED or FHIR's resource definitions), and organizational interoperability (the overarching legal, policy, and trust frameworks), enabling the effective cross-border application of these technical standards [19]. Common standards such as the European Electronic Health Record Exchange Format (EEHRxF) will be crucial.

In view of the current highly fragmented European healthcare landscape, it is by no means trivial for the players in the healthcare industry, both from an organizational and technological point of view, to offer solutions for hospitals and doctors that interact in a meaningful way without changing the content of data. On the one hand, the aforementioned common rules and standards for ensuring syntactic and semantic interoperability must be defined and monitored within the EHDS framework and governance structures, and, on the other hand, it must remain affordable to meet these requirements, especially for smaller players such as startups and medium-sized companies. To support this, the Commission launched the HealthData@EU central platform, released as open source in March 2025 [20]. It provides a catalogue, gateway services, and interoperability components for the secondary use of health data across Member States.

Without interoperability, it will not be possible to achieve a target-oriented holistic use of the data in question. The envisaged "single market" may perhaps be even more important for smaller countries than is currently the case from a point of view of larger countries like Germany, France, Italy or Poland; however, it is clear that a knowledge and technological advantage for each country's players in this field is completely unthinkable at the global level if the existing patchwork of different systems from electronic health records and hospital information systems to biobanks and research databases is not overcome as quickly as possible. Theoretically, telemedicine services should also be offered across borders. There will only be the best solutions for patients if the data allows for it. Pilot initiatives such as the EHDS2 Project (2022–2024) and TEHDAS2 Joint Action tested cross-border technical solutions, interoperability, and governance models. Their outcomes informed the regulation's technical and governance framework [21].

7.5 Clear Legislation avoiding Overlaps and Over-Regulation to simplify Compliance

Clarity will be essential in the interplay between the EHDS and related legislation. The "unleashing of the European data economy" can only be possible through a digital transformation of Europe into a digital single market. However, especially regarding the commercialization of digital health solutions, there are still insurmountable obstacles. In the fast-growing field of digital health, innovators often face major barriers to entry, as regulatory, reimbursement, and procurement processes across Europe are highly fragmented and difficult to tap. Such barriers delay patients' and citizens' access to effective solutions. The legal complexity and overlaps with other regulations affecting the healthcare sector—such as the "Medical Device Regulation," "Health Technology Assessment Regulation," and the EU "AI Act"—must be carefully aligned to avoid the risk of over-regulation. Legislation must be clear and user-friendly for both innovators and early adopters of modern technologies, both on European and in member state levels. Nevertheless, in view of the established but incompatible hospital information and practice management systems, decisive political alignment and prioritization will be required to achieve interoperability across legacy systems. Only if a maximum of the amount of data available under the European umbrella is available for both patients and innovators can we do justice to the pioneering roles that Germany and France have taken on through the Digital Care Act and the associated entitlement of insured persons to benefits and reimbursement for the supply of digital health applications (DiGA and PECAN).

The EHDS will roll out in phases. By March 2027, Member States must designate Health Data Access Bodies (HDABs), which will be fully operational by March 2029 to facilitate regulated access to health data for secondary use. But not every member state has reached the same level of progress. In Estonia for example, a pioneer in digital governance, the Estonian Health and Welfare Information Systems Centre (TEHIK) with its origins tracing back to the early 2000s with the development of the e-Health record system still has no final clarity on their institutional role under the EHDS. In France, on the other hand, the Health Data Hub was officially established in 2019 with the mission to facilitate access to health data for research and innovation and is well equipped to take on the role as a HDAB. In Germany, the Forschungsdatenzentren (Research Data Centres) have been created as foreseen in the Health Data Use Act (GDNG), which was adopted in 2024. HDABs will be able to grant permits for access to health datasets according to standard processes. Also by 2029, the first priority categories of data (e.g., patient summaries, electronic prescriptions) must be exchangeable under the rules for primary use. By 2031, additional categories will follow, broadening the scope of both primary and secondary uses. To operationalize the regulation, over 20 implementing acts are planned, covering technical standards, interoperability, privacy, cybersecurity, and procedures for granting access [22].

The bottom line is that the EU Commission has now presented clear conditions and created a suitable legal framework. Now it is up to the Member States to gain trust in society on the one hand and to create technological conditions on the other. The fact that neither will be an easy undertaking has already been shown in the recent past. Public skepticism toward data sharing underscores the need for proactive trust-building and communication strategies. The example of the large crowd of vaccine sceptics, who were hardly open to scientific arguments during the COVID pandemic and in many cases tended to fall prey to conspiracy theories, gives an idea of the resistance to alleged “data theft” that could still be expected. Indeed, progress will depend on better coordination, shared standards, and cultural change across the health sector [23]. Local pilot projects, clear legal frameworks, incentives for data sharing, and stronger communication will build trust and make the EHDS work in real-world settings [24].

The enforcement of the EHDS Regulation may be difficult considering the current diverse national realities across Member States [25].

Member States must now establish interoperable infrastructures that combine security, usability, and cross-border functionality—a goal previously pursued primarily by private technology firms: powerful cloud or crowd systems that not only secure the data in the background but also make it usable across systems and borders, while on the user side, the operation is as simple, attractive, and clear as possible so that digital health can actually find its way into the real life of each individual.

References

1. Hoeller K. EHDS – Der Europäische Gesundheitsdatenraum (Was Europa und die Mitgliedsstaaten jetzt tun müssen), vol. 94. München: Hanns-Seidel-Stiftung e.V.; 2023. p. 34–43. Accessed: 10 Oct 2025. [Online]. Available: https://www.hss.de/publikationen/ehds-der-europaeische-gesundheitsdatenraum-pub2416/.
2. European Union. Regulation (EU) 2016/679 of the European Parliament and of the Council. Europa.eu. Apr 27, 2016. https://eur-lex.europa.eu/eli/reg/2016/679/oj/eng.
3. von der Leyen U. Mission Letter for the Appointment of Stella Kyriakides as Commissioner for Health and Food Safety. Dec 2019. Accessed: 11 Oct 2025. [Online]. Available: https://commissioners.ec.europa.eu/system/files/2022-11/mission-letter-stella-kyriakides_en.pdf.
4. European Commission. A European Strategy for Data. Europa.eu. 2020. https://eur-lex.europa.eu/legal-content/EN/TXT/?qid=1582218646923&uri=COM:2020:66:FIN (Accessed 10 Oct 2025).
5. Schmidt L, Pawlitzki M, Renard BY, Meuth SG, Masanneck L. The three-year evolution of Germany's Digital Therapeutics reimbursement program and its path forward. npj Digit Med. 2024;7(1). https://doi.org/10.1038/s41746-024-01137-1.
6. Ministère du Travail, de la Santé, des Solidarités et des Familles. Le remboursement des thérapies numériques par l'Assurance maladie dans le cadre de la prise en charge anticipée numérique (PECAN) précisé – Ministère du Travail, de la Santé, des Solidarités et des Familles, sante.gouv.fr. May 02, 2024. https://sante.gouv.fr/actualites-presse/presse/communiques-de-presse/article/le-remboursement-des-therapies-numeriques-par-l-assurance-maladie-dans-le-cadre.
7. European Commission. Proposal for a Regulation of the European Parliament and of the Council on the European Health Data Space. May 03, 2022. https://health.ec.europa.eu/system/files/2022-05/com_2022-197_en.pdf (Accessed 11 Oct 2025).
8. Council of the European Union. European Health Data Space: council agrees its position. Council of the EU – Press Release. Dec 06, 2023. https://www.consilium.europa.eu/en/press/press-releases/2023/12/06/european-health-data-space-council-agrees-its-position/ (Accessed 11 Oct 2025).
9. Council of the European Union. European Health Data Space: Council and Parliament strike deal. Council of the EU – Press Release. Mar 15, 2024. https://www.consilium.europa.eu/en/press/press-releases/2024/03/15/european-health-data-space-council-and-parliament-strike-provisional-deal/ (Accessed 11 Oct 2025).
10. Official Journal of the European Union. Regulation (EU) 2025/327 of the European Parliament and of the Council of 11 February 2025 on the European Health Data Space and amending Directive 2011/24/EU and Regulation (EU) 2024/2847. 2025. Available: https://eur-lex.europa.eu/eli/reg/2025/327/oj/eng.
11. Directorate-General for Health and Food Safety (European Commission). European Health Data Space. Publications Office of the EU. 2023. https://op.europa.eu/en/publication-detail/-/publication/f2580615-8820-11ee-99ba-01aa75ed71a1/language-en# (Accessed 11 Oct 2025).
12. EU Directorate-General for Communication. Press Corner Questions and Answers – EU Health: European Health Data Space (EHDS). European Commission. May 03, 2022. https://ec.europa.eu/commission/presscorner/detail/en/qanda_22_2712.

13. Communication from the Commission to the European Parliament and the Council. A European Health Data Space: harnessing the power of health data for people, patients and innovation. May 2022. Accessed: 11 Oct 2025. [Online]. Available: https://health.ec.europa.eu/document/download/17c7065c-c432-445f-9b27-8ccf283581bc_en?filename=com_2022-196_en.pdf.
14. Federal Ministry for Economic Affairs and Energy (BMWi and Federal Ministry of Education and Research (BMBF). Project GAIA-X – A Federated Data Infrastructure as the Cradle of a Vibrant European Ecosystem. Oct 2019. Accessed: 11 Oct 2025. [Online]. Available: https://www.bundeswirtschaftsministerium.de/Redaktion/EN/Publikationen/Digitale-Welt/project-gaia-x.pdf?__blob=publicationFile&v=2.
15. Raab R, et al. Federated electronic health records for the European Health Data Space. Lancet Digit Health. 2023;5(11):e840–7. https://doi.org/10.1016/S2589-7500(23)00156-5.
16. EU Directorate-General for Health and Food Safety. Electronic cross-border health services. EU Public Health. Mar 05, 2025. https://health.ec.europa.eu/ehealth-digital-health-and-care/digital-health-and-care/electronic-cross-border-health-services_en (Accessed 11 Oct 2025).
17. EIT Health e.V. Learning from Health Data Use Cases – Real-world Challenges and Enablers to the Creation of the European Health Data Space. Nov 2021. Available: https://eithealth.eu/wp-content/uploads/2021/11/EHDS_report.pdf.
18. EIT Health e.V. EIT Health Statement on the European Health Data Space. May 2022. Accessed: 11 Oct 2025. [Online]. Available: https://eithealth.eu/wp-content/uploads/2022/05/EIT-Health-Statement-on-the-EHDS-proposal_final-05052022.pdf.
19. EU4Digital. Common Guidelines for eHealth Harmonisation and Interoperability. Europa.eu. Dec 2020. https://capacity4dev.europa.eu/library/common-guidelines-ehealth-harmonisation-and-interoperability_en.
20. European Union. HealthData@EU Central Platform. Europa.eu. 2025. https://acceptance.data.health.europa.eu/healthdata-central-platform?locale=en (Accessed 11 Oct 2025).
21. European Health and Digital Executive Agency (HaDEA). EU-funded projects contributing to the implementation of the European Health Data Space. EU News Article. Mar 28, 2025. https://hadea.ec.europa.eu/news/eu-funded-projects-contributing-implementation-european-health-data-space-2025-03-28_en.
22. European Commission Directorate-General for Health and Food Safety. European Health Data Space Regulation (EHDS). Public Health. Mar 05, 2025. https://health.ec.europa.eu/ehealth-digital-health-and-care/european-health-data-space-regulation-ehds_en (Accessed 11 Oct 2025).
23. Wilkesmann J, Höckel K, Höller K. Implementing the European Health Data Space in Germany & Switzerland Vol. 1: partners and experts perspective. Göttingen: © CUVILLIER VERLAG; 2023. Accessed: 11 Oct 2025. [Online]. Available: https://www.researchgate.net/publication/394884188_Implementing_the_European_Health_Data_Space_in_Germany_Switzerland_Vol_1_Partners_and_Experts_Perspective.
24. Wilkesmann J, Höckel K, Morales E, Walter L, Höller K. Recommendations for Further Action when Implementing the European Health Data Space in Germany. 2024. Available: https://www.researchgate.net/publication/394886445_Recommendations_for_Further_Action_when_Implementing_the_European_Health_Data_Space_in_Germany.
25. EIT Health e.V. Implementing the European Health Data Space across Europe. EIT Health Think Tank. 2024. https://eithealth.eu/think-tank-topic/implementing-the-european-health-data-space/.

Part III

Frameworks and Strategies for the Adoption of Digital Health in Clinical Practice

8 Adoption Frameworks for Digital Health Solutions in Hospital Settings

Andreas Lange

8.1 Integration of Digital Health into Clinical Workflows and Hospital IT Systems

With the commitment of IT departments and the financial support structure provided by the Hospital Future Act (KHZG), many hospitals in Germany have taken an important step toward digital solutions. The second DigitalRadar survey from June 2024 shows an increase in the average DigitalRadar score from 33.3 to 42.4 points, an increase of 9.1 points or 27.3%. Particularly significant improvements were seen in the areas of "Structures and Systems," "Clinical Processes," and "Information Exchange." This shows that KHZG funding has led to measurable progress [1].

While significant progress has already been made within individual hospitals, cross-institutional or cross-sectoral cooperation with digital solutions remains a particular challenge, as the following section will examine in more detail.

An international comparison shows that Germany lags behind countries such as Denmark, Estonia, and Canada in terms of the degree of digitization in its hospitals. For example, German hospitals only achieve a median score of 3 out of 7 in the international HIMSS-EMRAM model, while Scandinavian countries and the Netherlands have significantly higher maturity levels. OECD indicators on the use of electronic patient records and digital care processes also show that the pace of digitization is slower in Germany. These comparisons highlight the need to catch up, particularly with regard to standardized processes, end-to-end interoperability, and strategic coordination across institutions and sectors.

The following sections examine how these developments are reflected in organization, technology, infrastructure, and acceptance.

A. Lange (✉)
Klinik IT eG, Munich, Germany
e-mail: a.lange@klinik-it.de

S. Scholz et al. (eds.), *Advancements in Digital Health and Care*,
https://doi.org/10.1007/978-3-032-16837-5_8

8.1.1 Organizational Integration and Change Management

Digital healthcare solutions must be seamlessly integrated into existing clinical workflows in order to gain acceptance and achieve efficiency gains [2]. Due to the heterogeneity of hospital services and departments, it is essential that the technology be adapted to local processes [3]. Many hospitals are currently discussing the extent to which existing processes actually need to be customized. These special features are often rooted in the organizational structure and history of the respective institution. From an IT perspective, however, many of these processes can be standardized without restricting medical practice or clinical freedom of decision-making. Rather, the aim is to create a regulated and transparent organizational structure that can also be adapted to new digital tools and systems within the framework of well-managed change management. Early involvement of all stakeholders (including doctors, nursing staff, IT) and professional change management are critical success factors in reducing resistance [4]. Studies emphasize that a clear, communicated vision and buy-in from staff are crucial for successful change.

However, surveys in European hospitals show that change management methods are still not used systematically enough (implementation gap), which underscores the need to firmly anchor change management in the organizational culture [5]. At the same time, it can be observed that in some hospitals, committed actors in management structures are setting out to develop new and context-appropriate approaches to change management that question existing routines and establish creative forms of participation and communication. If standardized processes and clear procedures were established in hospital structures beforehand, digital projects could be implemented much more easily and quickly. In addition, IT specialists would be significantly relieved of work with, as they currently spend a large part of their time bridging ambiguities in organizational processes (who is the responsible process owner and has the authority to redesign this process) before new solutions can even be implemented. It would therefore be ideal if every IT project were preceded by an upstream organizational project that first clarifies processes, roles, and standards.

In hospitals, the "organizational project" is a focused 4- to 8-week pre-implementation track that stabilizes care processes before any configuration begins. A cross-functional team (clinicians, nursing, pharmacy, operations, IT) uses Lean value-stream mapping from admission to discharge to surface handoffs and waste, frames priority workflows with SIPOC (e.g., e-medication, discharge planning, OR scheduling), clarifies decision rights via a RACI, and agrees minimum viable standards for data and controls (dose units, allergy codes, patient identifiers, order-set naming, barcode conventions, audit trails). The track also fixes the operating model, process owners, governance cadence, KPIs, and standard work and converts results into a costed backlog for the build plus a change plan tied to measurable process targets.

For example, before introducing an e-medication module, a hospital runs a six-week organizational track to harmonize order sets, clarify ward–pharmacy handoffs, and set metrics for turnaround time and error rates. When the IT project begins, configuration and training focus on these agreed standards, reducing rework and accelerating adoption because roles, rules, and data are already settled.

On this basis, digital solutions could be implemented in a targeted and efficient manner, rather than simply electrifying existing, potentially inefficient processes. Both in corporate structures at larger institutions and in IT collaborations that extend beyond individual institutions, it is clear that standardization is also possible across institutions. Practical experience, for example, from the cooperation between the Diak Clinic in Schwäbisch Hall and the Crailsheim Clinic or the cooperation between Southeast Bavaria and InnKlinikum, shows that such harmonization is not only feasible from a technological standpoint or within a single institution but also depends significantly on the commitment and cooperation of the parties involved.

Organizational clarity is a prerequisite for successful technical integration, as described in the following section.

8.1.2 Technical Integration and Interoperability

Connecting new digital tools to existing hospital IT (e.g., HIS) requires standardized interfaces and data formats. In Germany, the use of open, international standards (e.g., HL7/FHIR for clinical data or DICOM for image data) is required by law to achieve end-to-end interoperability. Sections 371–375 of SGB V in conjunction with Section 19 KHG and Section 68 SGB V require hospitals to only use IT systems with standardized interfaces that have been approved by gematik [6]. Accordingly, the ISiK (Information Exchange in Hospitals) interoperability initiative was launched, which is based on HL7 FHIR. This initiative defines uniform APIs so that new applications (e.g., mobile visit apps, decision support systems) can communicate seamlessly with the HIS. All important German e-health specifications, from medical information objects (MIOs) to telematics infrastructure, are currently based on FHIR R4 (version 4.0.1), which promotes compatibility between systems [7].

ISiK is only a first step toward standardized communication within inpatient care. Initiatives such as ISiP (information exchange in cross-sector care) are currently being prepared for further development toward a cross-sector digital health infrastructure. At the same time, MIOs (medical information objects) are being developed for cross-sector applications, for example, in nursing communication or in connecting rehabilitation and general practices. These developments show that interoperability is not only a technical task but also a strategic one that must be continuously adapted to new care contexts and stakeholders.

However, what appears convincing in theory often encounters considerable obstacles in practice. Although the manufacturers of primary systems have obtained certification on time, the actual implementation and market availability of the specified interfaces are limited or come at high cost [8]. This is particularly critical when only a few of the connected subsystems (such as RIS, LIS, PACS) actually support the new standards: the effort required for implementation in the first use cases is enormous, while the immediate additional benefits are limited. Against this backdrop, many hospitals, especially in the current economic situation, are shying away from the necessary investments, especially since the added value can often only be demonstrated in the long term in a business case [9].

To make the long-term value visible, hospitals can use a lightweight benefits-realization approach anchored in the Quadruple Aim. Define a small, stable set of indicators, clinical outcomes (e.g., adverse drug-event rate, guideline adherence, length of stay), patient experience (PROMs/PREMs), workforce impact (minutes per task, overtime, turnover/burnout proxy), and financials (cost per case, avoided spend, NPV/ROI). Baseline these before go-live, set target deltas and time-to-benefit, and track adoption and process capability alongside them, so early leading indicators can validate the business case before lagging savings appear.

For example, for an e-medication rollout, the benefits register sets a 30% reduction in prescribing errors, pharmacy verification ≤15 min, barcode-scan compliance ≥85% by month six, a 0.2-day LOS reduction for selected DRGs, and 20 min per nurse per shift saved. Using agreed unit costs, the program reports value-on-investment in year one and a positive three-year NPV, making the long-term case auditable.

The MII's data integration centers (DIZ) use standardized FHIR-based models to demonstrate how structured data integration works in practice. These experiences offer valuable lessons learned for broader implementation in non-university hospitals [10]. However, hospitals generally lack the necessary technical infrastructure, suitable interfaces, specific expertise, or simply the human resources to implement these solutions on site [11]. In addition to syntax standards, semantic interoperability is also gaining in importance: the use of uniform terminology (e.g., SNOMED CT for diagnoses, LOINC for laboratory data) ensures that exchanged information is understood in the same way by all systems. Such standards and interfaces should be integrated into the hospital's IT strategy at an early stage in order to integrate digital solutions smoothly and avoid isolated solutions [12].

8.1.3 IT Infrastructure and Security Fundamentals

A robust digital infrastructure is essential for successful integration. Hospitals need high-performance networks, available server/cloud resources, and support structures to operate new digital services (such as telemedicine or AI tools) on a permanent basis. At the same time, high data protection and information security requirements must be taken into account, as health data is particularly sensitive [11]. The IT security strategy must be an integral part of digitization projects from the outset. In Germany, hospitals (above a certain size) are considered critical infrastructure with legal requirements under the IT Security Act and § 75c of the Sozialgesetzbuch V (SGB V) or § (new) 391 SGB V: they must comply with the "state of the art" in IT security and demonstrate this regularly [13]. The industry-specific security standards (B3S Hospital) of the German Hospital Association define recognized catalogs of measures to ensure the availability, confidentiality, and integrity of hospital data. These include, for example, the operation of an information security management system (ISMS) in accordance with ISO 27001, 24/7 monitoring for cyber attacks, emergency plans, and access control concepts [14]. The Hospital Future Act (KHZG) already stipulated that at least 15% of funding must be spent on IT security. A secure, high-performance IT infrastructure is therefore a fundamental technical prerequisite for the integration of digital solutions. It ensures that digital processes function reliably and that patient trust is maintained through data protection (critical success factor) [15]. At the same time, most hospitals face enormous challenges: the average German hospital has only around 250 beds and fewer than ten IT employees. Despite legal requirements and financial support, it is almost impossible for individual clinics to meet the high requirements of information security and digital operations management on their own, even with considerable effort [16]. Within hospital groups, attempts are therefore being made to pool synergies. A new and promising approach is the cross-institutional merger of smaller hospitals or networks—such as the Klinik IT eG model—to jointly meet requirements and develop and share resources, expertise, and infrastructure in the form of a cooperative [17].

8.1.4 AI Readiness and Advanced Technologies

With the increasing importance of artificial intelligence in healthcare, hospitals must also create the conditions for AI-based solutions. This includes not only technical aspects such as sufficient computing capacity and structured data sets but also ethical guidelines and governance structures for the responsible use of AI [18]. However, we are only at the beginning of this development: the necessary governance structures are established in very few hospitals and certainly not across different institutions if shared technology is to be used in care networks. Perhaps this is one of the reasons why AI solutions have been slow to find their way into everyday hospital practice. In addition, almost every manufacturer now advertises AI components, but rarely clarifies whether they involve rule-based process automation, machine learning, or generative AI, for example.

To make this concrete, AI in hospitals already covers distinct families: rule-based automation in clinical decision support (drug–drug and allergy checks, renal dosing, sepsis bundles) and administrative workflows (coding and claims edits); classical machine learning for risk prediction and operations (early sepsis and deterioration alerts, readmission and length-of-stay forecasts, patient-flow, and staffing forecasts); deep-learning pattern recognition in imaging and pathology (triage and prioritization, fracture and stroke detection, nodule sizing, digital slide classification); and generative/NLP systems that draft notes, discharge summaries and patient letters, extract data from free text, and support ambient documentation. Surgical platforms increasingly blend computer vision and planning with constrained autonomy for tasks such as instrument tracking or suture assistance. Being explicit about which family is used matters, because the data requirements, validation methods, explainability, and regulatory pathways differ and so do the expected benefits and risks.

The term "AI" is increasingly being used as a marketing term, but there is often a lack of clear differentiation between technical approaches. This leads to further uncertainty, ambiguity, and reluctance to use AI. The integration of AI systems therefore requires not only technical excellence but also education, differentiation, and clear governance with regard to the intended use, data basis, and responsibility [19].

AI governance in the hospital context is the regulatory framework of the European Union, in particular Regulation (EU) 2024/1206 on artificial intelligence (AI Act). This regulation establishes a binding set of rules for high-risk AI systems, which include numerous applications in healthcare, and formulates requirements for transparency, risk management, data quality, and internal control mechanisms. Compliance with these requirements is essential for the development of viable governance structures in hospitals, particularly with regard to clarifying legal responsibilities, auditability, and traceability of algorithmic decisions.

Another key ethical aspect concerns the need for a structured approach to potential bias, validation, and auditing of AI applications. For responsible and accepted use in clinical practice, AI systems must be designed to be transparent, non-discriminatory, and systematically verifiable, especially with regard to their role in diagnostic decisions or clinical decision support. Regulation (EU) 2024/1206 (AI Act) also contains clear requirements in this regard, for example on risk assessment, documentation of training data, and the establishment of independent review mechanisms. These requirements should be an integral part of every AI strategy in hospitals and serve as the ethical and legal basis for trustworthy AI use.

Analogous to established maturity models such as HIMSS-EMRAM or the German DigitalRadar, the maturity level of AI could also be systematically recorded and evaluated. Such a classification for example, along the dimensions of data availability, algorithmic transparency, clinical integration, regulatory compliance, and ethical evaluation, could help hospitals realistically assess their status and derive targeted development steps. In the long term, it would be desirable to integrate a standardized "AI Readiness Index" into existing maturity models to enable strategic assessment and comparability in a national and international context. This would include structured data, computing power, and ethical and organizational frameworks.

8.2 Overcoming Implementation Barriers: Case Studies and Solutions

8.2.1 Overcoming Human and Organizational Hurdles

The introduction of digital innovations often fails less because of technology than because of cultural barriers in hospitals. Resistance arises, for example, when employees fear additional work or a loss of quality. A practical example from a case study shows that the perception and benefits of the technology must be clearly recognizable to clinical staff, otherwise the relative advantage over old methods remains questionable. Solutions lie in change management: training and early involvement make employees feel empowered rather than threatened [4]. A multinational study recommended clear communication of the vision for change, involvement of all professional groups from the outset, and adaptation to the local work culture as factors for success [5]. In addition, some clinics are starting to consistently pursue lean hospital approaches. In combination with and upstream of digitization projects, this methodology has shown in practice that digital projects can be implemented much more quickly and stringently [20]. International best practices demonstrate successful approaches: in Estonia, a national digitization strategy and consistent citizen participation have achieved an electronic health record usage rate of over 99% [21]. Denmark relied on regional pilot projects with intensive user involvement before introducing national standards. Finland combined strong political leadership with bottom-up innovations from the field. In the past, German hospitals have sometimes lacked such systematic change management, which is why change agents or digital multipliers are important in teams to serve as multipliers. Managers should also make successes visible early on (quick wins) to convince skeptical employees. Case studies from the COVID-19 pandemic show that committed leadership and interdisciplinary collaboration can significantly accelerate digital transformation [4]. Against this backdrop, the hospital reform that came into force on January 1, 2025, is also of particular importance: The legal provisions of the Hospital Care Improvement Act (KHVVG) aim to ensure that individual clinics not only organize themselves better but also establish cross-institutional and cross-sector care networks. This is precisely why the implementation of systematic change management is crucial, both for cross-functional digital projects and for issues relating to joint patient care. This requirement has not yet been recognized in many hospitals, as they are initially preoccupied with classification into care levels, securing budgets, and the remaining funding opportunities. The necessary IT infrastructures and interoperable system landscapes have also often not yet been recognized as strategic prerequisites. Overall, the following applies: organization-wide digital literacy, interprofessional cooperation, and an open error culture promote the sustainable implementation of new applications.

8.2.2 Technical Integration Problems and Legacy Systems

The established IT landscape is often a major obstacle: hospital systems are historically heterogeneous and fragmented, which makes it difficult to introduce new digital tools. Case studies show that innovations in hospitals can fail if they cannot be integrated into various departments and existing software environments [22]. Legacy systems are often monolithic legacy HIS with proprietary interfaces. Lessons learned from failed projects reveal typical sources of error: underestimating the complexity of existing systems, failing to involve the IT department from the outset, lacking test phases, and inadequate data migration plans. According to a recent study, inadequate technical preparation and lack of integration were the reasons for around 60% of digitalization projects that were not successfully completed

[23]. Creating interoperability and migration architectures is therefore key to overcoming technical barriers. Solutions include the use of middleware or integration platforms and the consistent use of standardized interfaces (see 8.1.2). In Germany, structural solutions have been created to remove technical barriers through legal requirements (Sections 371–375 of the German Social Code, Book V) and programs such as ISiK. For example, in the past, hospitals had to develop individual interfaces for each device manufacturer; now, a FHIR-based exchange format is intended to facilitate the connection of new systems to the HIS [24]. However, practical experience shows that many software manufacturers only make these standardized interfaces available to hospitals to a limited extent or at high costs. As a result, the potential benefits of standardization often fall short of expectations in practice. Several initiatives are therefore currently underway in Germany to create platforms that will enable truly interoperable data exchange across institutions and sectors. As the implementation of legal requirements is repeatedly delayed, hospital initiatives are launching pragmatic initiatives to set up their own platforms, which can be replaced by legally regulated solutions in the future, provided that these actually fulfill the practical needs of hospitals. Examples include the Mein-Krankenhaus. Digital project by Klinik IT eG in Munich, the Gesundheitsplattform Rheinland-Pfalz, Health Harbour Hamburg, and the cooperation between Charité and Vivantes in Berlin. However, hospital groups and individual hospitals are also going their own way, such as Alexianer, Helios, Asklepios, and Sana Kliniken. Integration profiles from IHE (Integrating the Healthcare Enterprise) are also being used in isolated cases to exchange laboratory findings or medication data between systems, for example. Another obstacle is the lack of interoperability between sectors (outpatient and inpatient). In Germany, data exchange platforms such as the telematics infrastructure (TI) are being expanded so that referrals, emergency data, and e-prescriptions, for example, can be transferred seamlessly and without media breaks between systems.

8.2.3 Data Protection, Regulation, and Financing

Strict data protection requirements (EU GDPR, national law) can delay the implementation of digital solutions. In Germany, trust in digital health solutions is closely linked to data security. According to the Charité, particular emphasis is placed on ensuring that patient privacy is the top priority whenever digital cloud solutions are introduced [25]. However, an international comparison reveals a different trend: in many countries, a pragmatic assessment is made of the specific benefits that digital health applications bring to patients and how these can be reconciled with appropriate data protection standards. In the German debate, therefore, a critical assessment must be made of whether patients benefit more from the protection of their data or from the effective, interoperable exchange of this information in the interests of better healthcare. For example, health data may only be stored on servers that meet the high requirements of the BSI; this often excludes the use of non-European cloud services or requires technically complex measures (encryption, pseudonymous storage, dedicated data centers). A case study on the introduction of electronic patient records (ePA) in Germany highlights regulatory hurdles: unclear access rights for those involved and a lack of emergency provisions in the event of IT failures contributed to the delay, as did insufficient communication about the benefits and handling of the ePA [26]. Solutions include further development of the legal framework; for example, an opt-out solution for ePA was introduced in January 2025 to increase the usage rate, accompanied by clearer guidelines on consent and access logs [27]. On the other hand, transparent communication strategies are needed: international experience (e.g., Estonia, Denmark) shows that broad public education about the added value of digital files and high security standards increase trust [28]. In addition to data protection, financial aspects also pose an obstacle: the introduction of a clinical decision support system, for example, requires considerable investment without any immediate return on investment. However, the connection of these decision support systems is technically complex, and the benefits would initially be felt primarily in the quality of care. This quality feature is only rudimentarily taken into account in the German hospital remuneration system, which does not make the economic decision easy for hospitals currently in a difficult financial situation [9]. In Germany, this barrier has been partially addressed by funding programs such as the Hospital Future Fund (KHZF, €4.3 billion) and the Innovation Fund (€200 million annually for healthcare research). Hospitals were able to apply for earmarked grants for digital projects, which enabled best practice projects (e.g., digital patient portals, telemedicine platforms). However, one condition was always co-financing and a commitment to continue operating from their own resources after the funding ended which poses challenges for smaller hospitals [29]. One solution here is to develop sustainability plans at an early stage: financing, operation, and scaling should be considered for the long term right from the pilot phase of digital projects. Studies show that clear legal frameworks, binding standardization requirements, and financial incentives can make a significant contribution to overcoming implementation barriers. In addition, innovative financing models should also be considered, such as pay-for-performance approaches, earmarked innovation budgets, or targeted DRG surcharges for digital infrastructure. Such mechanisms could create targeted incentives for quality-oriented and sustainable digitization.

8.2.4 Patient Perspective and Acceptance

Societal acceptance of digital health solutions is a key prerequisite for their successful implementation and sustainable use. Patients are not only the target group but also active participants in the digital transformation, their perspective is a decisive factor in the success of technological innovations in the healthcare context.

A key influencing factor that has received too little attention to date is patient acceptance of digital health solutions. Studies show that patient trust and engagement are crucial for the sustainable use of digital services.

Key aspects of patient acceptance can be structured along technological, communicative, and normative dimensions:

- Technological dimension: User-friendliness is essential, especially for people who are less tech-savvy. Systems must be intuitive to use and provide barrier-free interfaces. This is particularly important for vulnerable groups such as older people, people with disabilities, or people with limited language skills. The requirements of EU Directive 2019/882 on the accessibility of digital products provide a key reference framework in this regard.
- Communicative dimension: Patients want transparent information about the use of their health data, including the ability to access it at any time. Concrete benefits—such as faster transmission of findings or the avoidance of duplicate examinations—must be communicated clearly and comprehensively.
- Normative dimension: Preserving data sovereignty is central to many users. They want to determine for themselves who has access to their data and how it may be used.

The Patient Engagement Framework, which describes various levels of activation, from pure information to active participation in decisions is a useful conceptual framework. In addition, the WHO's definition of "digital health literacy" provides a normative framework for empowering patients to use digital services competently and independently.

The introduction of the opt-out ePA from 2025 marks a paradigm shift: instead of having to actively register, patients must now actively object. This requires particular sensitivity in health communication and comprehensive information campaigns to build trust and allay fears.

8.2.5 Perspective of Healthcare Professionals

The perspective of healthcare professionals is also a key factor in the success of digital transformation in hospitals. Studies show that doctors, nurses, and therapists are generally positive about digital technologies, provided that they lead to concrete improvements in their everyday work and are intuitive to use [30].

Typical barriers to acceptance vary between professional groups:

- Nurses report unclear roles when it comes to using digital tools, especially for maintaining master data or operating mobile documentation systems. On top of that, there are often extra documentation requirements with no real added value, plus a lot of time pressure when working shifts, which makes training and getting used to things harder.
- Medical staff, on the other hand, express reservations about the reliability and clinical relevance of digital decision-making aids, especially in AI-supported applications. There are also uncertainties regarding legal responsibility and liability for automated decisions, as well as concerns about additional administrative work.

Solutions lie in the early involvement of all professional groups, the provision of tailored training opportunities, and close coordination between IT, management, and hospital staff. Digital applications must be embedded not only technically but also in terms of work organization [31].

Experience from KHZG projects and international model clinics shows that when professionals experience noticeable relief, better information, and greater certainty in clinical decisions, acceptance also increases. Corresponding accompanying research emphasizes the importance of targeted change communication, feedback loops, and the identification of "digital champions" in order to anchor transformation processes in the long term. The continuous promotion of digital skills, for example, in the context of microlearning formats, simulation training, or interdisciplinary learning forums, is a cornerstone of long-term success.

8.2.6 Scaling and Transfer to Broad Healthcare Provision

Many digital solutions start as pilot projects, the challenge is to successfully scale them up to entire clinics or networks. This requires strategic planning that goes beyond the mere use of technology. Theoretical frameworks such as the NASSS framework (non-adoption, abandonment, scale-up, spread, sustainability) developed by Greenhalgh et al. provide guidance by highlighting relevant dimensions (from the clinical picture to technology and value propositions to organizational and market aspects) [32].

Compared to other models such as the Consolidated Framework for Implementation Research (CFIR), the RE-AIM framework, or the WHO Digital Health Atlas, NASSS stands out for its particular suitability for evaluating complex, long-term implementation projects in highly regulated healthcare structures. While CFIR primarily highlights internal implementation conditions and RE-AIM focuses on evaluation effects, NASSS explicitly integrates contextual dynamics and changeability over time. It thus offers a particularly practical framework for hospitals that want to develop data- and risk-based scaling and sustainability strategies.

The NASSS framework distinguishes seven key dimensions that influence the success or failure of digital innovations in healthcare:

- Condition: The more complex or unpredictable the course of a disease, the more difficult digitization is.
- Technology: Technical maturity, depth of integration, and usability influence acceptance and scalability. Modular architectures, multi-tenancy, and standard APIs are of central importance here.
- Value proposition: Innovation projects must deliver tangible added value for patients, healthcare professionals, and payers alike.
- Adopters: The willingness and ability of user groups to embrace new digital processes is crucial.
- Organization: Internal structures, culture, resources, and leadership play a key role in implementation.

- Infrastructure and regulation (Wider System): External conditions such as data protection, remuneration, and interoperability requirements also determine success.
- Embedding and adaptation over time: The ability to further develop and adapt innovations over time is central to sustainability.

The NASSS framework provides support in the scaling-up process in particular through its systematic analysis of scaling barriers. It reveals, for example, whether the solution is technologically robust but not organizationally compatible, or whether regulatory barriers are slowing down expansion. For hospitals, it thus provides a structured basis for decision-making (e.g., when choosing between centralized vs. decentralized rollout) in order to anticipate risks, derive targeted change measures, and plan implementation strategies realistically.

In practical terms, this means that process standardization and modular system architecture facilitate expansion to other departments or locations. Another critical success factor is the early involvement of hospital management and cost centers in order to plan the resources (budget, personnel) required for expansion.

Concrete implementation strategies such as the SmartHospital.NRW process model offer structured approaches for gradual scaling:

- Assessment phase: Determination of maturity level and analysis of current situation.
- Strategy development: Definition of digitization goals.
- Piloting: Small-scale tests with defined success criteria.
- Rollout: Gradual expansion with continuous monitoring.
- Optimization: Iterative improvement based on user feedback.

International comparisons show that successful scaling usually occurs where continuous performance measurement and feedback mechanisms have been established. For example, in a Canadian heart clinic, the telemonitoring service was iteratively adapted and expanded based on outcome data and user feedback until it became routine for thousands of patients [33, 34].

Standardized maturity models (such as HIMSS EMRAM or DigitalRadar Hospital) can help make digital progress measurable and identify gaps before large-scale rollout [35]. Nevertheless, there are few detailed publications in the literature on scientifically documented examples of successfully scaled digitization projects in hospital practice—a gap in the research [32].

To address this gap, future work should study the post-pilot scale-up with mixed-methods, multi-site, quasi-experimental designs. A pragmatic template is a stepped-wedge or difference-in-differences evaluation of staged roll-outs across hospitals, using a common outcome set aligned with the Quadruple Aim (clinical quality and safety, patient experience, workforce impact, and costs) plus leading indicators for adoption and process capability. Context should be captured with a NASSS-informed complexity profile and reported alongside time-to-value, total cost of ownership, and sustainability beyond initial funding, including neutral or negative results. An open registry of scaled implementations with standardized measures would enable cross-site learning and meta-analysis.

Decision-makers should therefore continue to apply proven change management practices (from 8.2.1) during the scaling phase: e.g., appoint key users in each department, plan step-by-step rollouts with sufficient training capacity, and communicate success stories to generate momentum for widespread adoption.

8.2.7 Interoperability and Standardization as the Basis for Sustainability

Interoperability across system and institutional boundaries is essential for the long-term success and future expansion of digital solutions. Only if new applications can exchange data with existing and future systems can they be embedded in larger care networks (horizontal scaling) and survive technology changes. Strategically, hospitals should therefore focus on open standards and actively participate in standardization initiatives.

One solution that hospitals should already be considering and incorporating into their standardization initiatives is the European Health Data Space (EHDS), which will be implemented in stages starting in March 2025. The EHDS creates:

- Uniform data formats for cross-border exchange.
- Common governance structures for secondary use of health data.
- Mandatory interoperability standards for all EU member states [36].

Strategic importance of the EHDS for hospitals.

The European Health Data Space (EHDS) is by no means primarily a research data project, but explicitly pursues a dual focus with equal importance for both patient care and research and innovation. The regulation distinguishes between two complementary forms of use:

Primary data use (direct care): treatment and rehabilitation, prescription and dispensing of medicines, continuity in cross-border care, access to electronic health records with patient summaries, e-prescriptions, medical images, and laboratory results

Secondary data use (research, innovation, policy-making): health research and product development, AI training, evaluation of digital health applications, public health monitoring, personalized care based on existing data

For primary use, the voluntary EU-wide infrastructure "MyHealth@EU," which enables cross-border data exchange, will be used. For secondary use, new national Health Data Access Bodies and the HealthData@EU platform will be established.

Another example of sustainability through standards is the national commitment to FHIR R4: All key projects, from ePA and e-prescriptions to research data sets from the Medical Informatics Initiative, use the same FHIR version, ensuring that interactions and updates can be controlled [37].

Semantic standards also contribute to future-proofing: The introduction of international medical terminologies (such as SNOMED CT, ICD-11, OPS, ATC) and mapping strategies between classifications enable clinical concepts to remain consistent even when applications change [38].

However, interoperability does not only mean technical connectivity, but also organizational connectivity, this includes standard processes for data exchange between sectors (e.g., hospital ↔ family doctor) and supraregional health data networks. One strategy is to establish so-called digital health ecosystems: platforms on which various actors (clinics, practices, research, public health) share data according to common rules [39].

It is crucial that clinics check compatibility and standards compliance for every new purchase. This foresight ensures that today's solutions can still be integrated tomorrow, rather than jeopardizing sustainability as technical debt.

8.2.8 Long-Term Viability and Continuous Improvement

Sustainability in clinical digital projects requires stable structures for operation and maintenance, on the one hand, and the ability to adapt to changing requirements, on the other. Governance models at the hospital, group, network, or cooperative level play a central role here, for example, digitization committees, CIO-led strategy rounds, or interdisciplinary innovation boards.

Clear processes are a decisive factor in the effective and rapid implementation of digital innovations in everyday hospital life. Without clearly defined responsibilities, decision-making paths, and procedures, many projects get stuck in the planning phase or lose momentum along the way. However, the pressure to digitize the healthcare sector is increasing, while technological possibilities are developing rapidly. To avoid falling behind internationally, hospitals must drastically shorten the duration of innovation cycles. This includes standardized procedures for assessing needs, agile project methods, and accelerated approval steps.

It is also important to integrate innovation processes with the reality of healthcare provision, for example, through the early involvement of users, testing in real clinical practice, and evaluation based on practical benefit criteria. Clear processes create trust and transparency, and enable scaling. They are therefore not an end in themselves, but one of the most effective levers for sustainable digital transformation.

A critical success factor is ongoing staff training: high turnover or new employees require continuous training to ensure that digital applications are used correctly and remain accepted. Studies emphasize that even well-established systems can lose their usefulness without regular refresher training and support [30]. Formats of lifelong (micro-)learning, continuously embedded digital learning impulses in everyday work, are becoming increasingly important. Structured mentoring programs can further enhance the effectiveness of learning processes.

It is equally important to establish adequate support, such as a 24/7 help desk or a super-user network—to quickly resolve everyday problems. As digital processes increasingly become critical components of care, a traditional on-call service is no longer sufficient in the event of problems. Instead, structures will have to be established that can provide adequate help and solutions consistently and systematically.

In addition, the provision of test systems in particularly critical areas is essential in order to be able to test new functions, configurations, or updates without risk before they are put into productive use. At the technical level, the maintainability of the systems must be guaranteed: this includes software updates, security patches, and the ability to add new functions in a modular fashion without jeopardizing the overall system operation.

Financial sustainability is also key: digital innovation must transition from project mode to routine operation. This requires continuous funding and organizational integration into the institution's standard processes. Successful clinics have institutionalized innovation boards, recurring retrospectives, and structured change management that views digitalization as an ongoing task. Business cases and benefit analyses have proven effective in convincing administrators and cost bearers of the need for long-term financing, for example, by demonstrating efficiency gains, quality improvements, or revenue increases in specific DRGs [9].

In practice, the business case that convinces boards pairs a total-cost-of-ownership and net-present-value view with a benefits register aligned to the Quadruple Aim. Productivity gains can be translated into avoided replacement costs/full-time equivalents, price certainty, and quality effects through avoided adverse events and readmissions; revenue gains can be quantified through complete coding, throughput, and fewer denials at the DRG-level; and, where applicable, the avoidance of risks/penatlies can be included. Where clinical outcomes are central or payer negotiations are in play, complement ROI with cost-effectiveness (e.g., incremental cost per QALY gained) to show value beyond internal savings. Track these benefits against a pre-go-live baseline with clear attribution rules, so finance sees value materializing over time.

For example, an outpatient clinic adopts an AI note assistant that cuts documentation time from 8 to 5 min per encounter. With 100 encounters per day over a period of 250 days, that amounts to 25,000 encounters and 75,000 minutes of time saved 1250 hours. At an all-in staff cost of €50/h, the annual benefit is ~€62,500. Costs are €35,000/year for licenses plus a one-off €20,000 setup. Year 1 net ≈ €7500; from Year 2 onward ≈ €27,500/year. Payback is roughly 11 months, with side benefits tracked via fewer documentation errors and higher staff satisfaction.

The clinic example above is the micro version of this board-ready logic: convert minutes saved into an annual avoided cost, place it in a three-year TCO/NPV view, then layer in safety/quality benefits as avoided events and DRG-level revenue lift; where clinical outcomes drive the case, add cost-effectiveness (e.g., € per QALY). Track all items against a pre-go-live baseline in a benefits register aligned with the Quadruple Aim so that payback and NPV become visible month by month.

In Germany, the introduction of reimbursable digital services (e.g., DiGA on prescription) has been a step toward economic sustainability. These digital health applications can be prescribed by physicians and reimbursed by statutory health insurance companies, which secures them a permanent place in standard care. No comparable structure exists for hospitals as yet: digital innovations such as patient portals, AI-based assistance systems, or digital pathway documentation are often only financed through temporary project budgets or special funding (e.g., KHZG). To ensure that these solutions do not expire at the end of the project, but can be operated, maintained, and further developed on a solid basis, reliable and predictable financing mechanisms are required within the framework of hospital remuneration. One possibility would be mandatory refinancing via DRG surcharges or flat-rate allowances for digital infrastructure [40].

Such structural anchoring would not only promote economic sustainability but also create an incentive for hospitals to invest in digital excellence. Cross-institutional initiatives, such as joint platform solutions or regionally coordinated data rooms, should also become eligible for funding and billing in the future. They not only enable economies of scale, but also strengthen cross-sector care and digital resilience in the healthcare system as a whole.

Finally, hospitals should focus on flexibility: the digital landscape is evolving rapidly (keywords: AI, IoT, personalized medicine). Sustainable strategies therefore involve adaptability—successful institutions create a culture of learning and adaptation. Pilot projects are deliberately kept small, but scaled up quickly if successful. This is precisely where a shortcoming in the German hospital system becomes apparent: innovation cycles are often too long to keep pace with the international speed of digital transformation. Procedures are complex, project approvals are lengthy, and decision-making processes are often too hierarchical to allow for rapid iterations.

That is why framework conditions are needed that allow successful solutions to be scaled up quickly, both within individual institutions and across different providers. This requires not only more courage to prioritize, but also adapted funding mechanisms, agile governance structures, and digital test environments with short response times. Cooperation models such as the medical informatics initiative with university data integration centers show how joint learning and coordinated action can accelerate this process [41].

Taking these factors into account, including institutional learning, feedback loops, governance, and user acceptance, significantly increases the chances of success for digital transformation.

References

1. DigitalRadar Hospital. Second survey 2024 – results and analyses. RWI – Leibniz Institute for Economic Research; 2024.
2. Wosny M, Strasser LM, Hastings J. JMIR Hum Factors. 2023;10:e50357.
3. Chambers DA, et al. Implement Sci. 2013;8:117.

4. Nilsen P, et al. BMC Health Serv Res. 2020;20:147.
5. Barrow JM, Annamaraju P. StatPearls. 2022.
6. Federal Ministry of Health. Law on the protection of electronic patient data in the telematics infrastructure (PDSG). BGBl I. 2020;(44):1879–92.
7. Gerloff R et al. (DKG). kma – IT & Digital Health. 2021.
8. Gehring T, Kiehntopf M, Prokosch HU. Challenges in the implementation of HL7 FHIR in German hospitals: a cross-sectional survey. Methods Inf Med. 2023;62(4):157–65.
9. Rau E, et al. Front Health Serv. 2024;4:1370759.
10. Medical Informatics Initiative. Press release MII research data portal. 2023.
11. German Hospital Institute (DKI). Study "The Digital Hospital." 2019.
12. Fung KW, Xu J, Bodenreider O. The role of standard terminologies in achieving semantic interoperability in healthcare. Yearb Med Inform. 2021;30(1):39–45.
13. German Hospital Association (DKG), implementation guidelines pursuant to Section 75c SGB V, 2021.
14. DKG & BSI. B3S Hospital Version 1.2. 2023.
15. Federal Ministry of Health (BMG). FAQ Hospital Future Act. 2020.
16. von Eiff W. Das Krankenhaus (The Hospital). 2023;115(5):404–7.
17. Klinik IT eG. https://klinik-it-eg.de/. Accessed July 2025.
18. World Health Organization (WHO). Ethics and governance of artificial intelligence for health. 2021.
19. American Medical Association (AMA). Establishing a governance framework for AI in health care. 2022.
20. Toussaint JS, Berry LL. The promise of lean in health care. Mayo Clin Proc. 2013;88(1):74–82.
21. OECD. Health at a glance: Europe 2022. Paris: OECD Publishing; 2022.
22. Torab-Miandoab A, et al. BMC Med Inform Decis Mak. 2023;23:18.
23. Torab-Miandoab A, Müller D, Esmailzadeh A, et al. Failure factors in hospital digitization: a mixed-methods review. BMC Med Inform Decis Mak. 2023;23:18.
24. Gematik. Interoperability portal – ISiK. 2022.
25. Bitkom e.V. Position paper on data protection in healthcare. 2020.
26. Schewior K, Schnell M. Introduction of the ePA in Germany: obstacles and lessons learned. Health Econ Qual Manag. 2024;29(3):102–9.
27. Federal Ministry of Health. gesund.bund.de – Electronic patient record. 2023.
28. Papadopoulos K, et al. Int J Public Health. 2024;69:1607288.
29. German Hospital Association (DKG). Hospital future fund: FAQ. 2020.
30. Antweiler D, et al. Bundesgesundheitsbl. 2024;67(1):66–75.
31. Greenhalgh T, Wherton J, Papoutsi C, et al. Beyond adoption: a new framework for theorizing and evaluating nonadoption, abandonment, and challenges to the scale-up, spread, and sustainability of health and care technologies. J Med Internet Res. 2017;19(11):e367.
32. Greenhalgh T, et al. Milbank Q. 2004;82(4):581–629.
33. Canada Health Infoway. Telemonitoring implementation report. 2022.
34. McGillion MH, et al. J Med Internet Res. 2021;23(9):e27328.
35. DigitalRadar Hospital. Methodology paper on maturity assessment. 2022.
36. European Commission. Proposal for a Regulation on the European Health Data Space. COM(2022) 197 final.
37. Medical Informatics Initiative. Research data portal – interoperability strategy. Berlin: TMF; 2023.
38. SNOMED International; WHO ICD-11; BfArM OPS classification; EMA ATC classification.
39. European Commission. EHDS project description. 2022.
40. German Hospital Federation (DKG). Position paper on digital infrastructure financing. Berlin; 2024.
41. Medical Informatics Initiative. Learning together, acting together: implementing data integration at university hospitals. Berlin: TMF; 2024.

Adoption Frameworks for Digital Health Solutions in Hospital Settings: Implementation Strategies from a Supplier Perspective

9

Janina Beilner and Kurt Höller

9.1 Introduction

The healthcare sector is undergoing a profound transformation driven by demographic shifts [1], rising patient expectations, sustainability imperatives, and financial pressures. Hospitals are increasingly expected to deliver high-quality care with fewer resources, while simultaneously improving operational efficiency, staff productivity, and environmental performance [2]. WHO projected a shortfall of 11 million health workers by 2030 [3]. This shortage underscores the need for digital health solutions that enhance efficiency and enable task-shifting while maintaining quality of care.

Initially, the concept of a "digital hospital" emerged, primarily focused on transitioning from paper-based systems to electronic health records (EHRs) [4]. As the focus broadened beyond mere digitization to encompass improved care, health outcomes, and cost reduction [5], the term "digital" started to evolve into "smart" [6], signaling a new era of integrating advanced technologies for more intelligent operations [7]. In context of this comprehensive data utilization and technological integration, the concept of the "smart hospital" has emerged as a strategic imperative.

Another increasingly vital dimension in the understanding of smart hospitals is their resilience. This perspective is notably championed by the Pan American Health Organization (PAHO), which has integrated its Smart Hospital project into the

J. Beilner (✉)
Healthcare Vertical Market, Siemens AG, Munich, Germany

Department of Artificial Intelligence in Biomedical Engineering, FAU Erlangen-Nuernberg, Erlangen, Germany
e-mail: janina.beilner@siemens.com

K. Höller
Healthcare Vertical Market, Siemens AG, Munich, Germany

CiNNAMED GmbH, Erlangen, Germany
e-mail: kurt.hoeller@siemens.com

S. Scholz et al. (eds.), *Advancements in Digital Health and Care*,
https://doi.org/10.1007/978-3-032-16837-5_9

broader Resilient Hospital program. PAHO defines a resilient hospital as "a safe, smart, and inclusive facility that is flexible and adaptable to transform and learn, through mitigation, preparedness, response, and recovery, within a multi-hazard approach and based on a strategic risk assessment" [8]. This definition expands the conventional view of hospitals, beyond their roles in public health, significant government expenditure, or CO_2 emissions, to recognize them as threatened critical infrastructure. Consequently, "smartness" and "flexibility" emerge as essential requirements for ensuring their resilience and preparedness against a multitude of hazards, including the latest potential threats such as geopolitical conflicts.

This chapter explores the frameworks and strategies for adopting digital health solutions in hospital settings, focusing on implementation from a supplier perspective.

9.2 The Case for Smart Hospitals

9.2.1 Four Steps to Becoming a Smart Hospital

Hospitals are facing diverse challenges such as aging populations, staff shortages, cost pressures, and sustainability demands. Traditional infrastructure is ill equipped to meet these evolving needs. A smart hospital offers a solution by integrating digital technologies to enhance patient outcomes, streamline operations, and reduce environmental impact.

Technically, smart hospitals are characterized by their robust data integration capabilities, enabling them to collect, analyze, and act on data from diverse sources, including clinical data from medical devices, administrative data from information technology infrastructure (IT), and building management data from operational technology systems (OT) [9]. This data-driven approach enables predictive maintenance, real-time asset tracking, personalized patient experiences, and optimized resource utilization. The transformation is not merely technological. It also represents a profound change management challenge affecting both organizational culture and operational processes. It requires rethinking of workflows, stakeholder engagement, and infrastructure design.

Digital technologies have quickly become an enabler for positive change within many different areas of healthcare and hospitals are no exception. Becoming a "smart hospital" has far reaching benefits from improved energy efficiency to reduced waste and increased staff productivity.

However, the digitalization of an entire hospital is a complex undertaking, and one that doesn't happen overnight. It is a journey with many steps along the way, but which is grounded in deploying future-proof technology that can adapt as tech naturally evolves.

9.2.1.1 Embarking on a Digital Revolution

Digitalization can automate and enhance many aspects of a hospital's infrastructure that impacts day-to-day operations across three main areas:

- Clinical operations, which can be improved by streamlining workflows, diagnostics and therapies which not only boosts staff productivity but has the potential to improve the delivery of healthcare services.
- Hospital operations, such as logistics and admin, which can be time consuming for staff and hinder their productivity.
- Building technology, which can manage the energy efficiency and automation of building structures, supporting cost and sustainability goals.

That last point—sustainability—is a critical driver for the digitalization of hospitals, as they currently account for ~5% of the world's carbon emissions [10]. Bringing that number down is a top concern for hospital CEOs.

In a compelling demonstration of energy efficiency, a study conducted in 2022 revealed that hospitals implementing AI systems for operating room optimization achieved a 25% reduction in energy consumption [3]. Another article states that AI is already helping companies reduce energy use by up to 60% [11]. This outcome highlights how comprehensive digitalization can significantly lower energy footprints across healthcare facilities, so that delivering great care doesn't come at the expense of the planet's finite resources. For all these reasons and more, digitalization is quickly becoming more than a "nice to have"; it's an essential travel companion on the road to net zero.

9.2.1.2 A Roadmap for Digitalization

One concern frequently mentioned is that people don't know where to start with digital transformation, and this is why that should be seen as a journey.

Traditionally, hospitals have been run in a way where buildings were operated reactively; solutions were based onsite; and control over the different elements, such as lighting, heating, and cooling, were siloed. Bringing all these operations together into one "smart" system would be difficult, as the building's infrastructure doesn't "talk" or feed into an integrated control system.

Stage 1: Connected Hospital

The first step from traditional to automated begins with getting connected by implementing basic sensor networks throughout the hospital facility. This means installing environmental sensors (temperature, humidity, air quality), occupancy sensors, and equipment monitors that can collect real-time data. Here it is key to prioritize sensors that integrate through shared and common protocols rather than "closed" or proprietary systems in order to ensure interoperability and limit interface costs.

Given the scale and complexity of hospital infrastructures, the initial implementation phase often appears challenging, so an important first step for a hospital would be to identify high-impact areas, e.g., operating theaters, patient rooms, pharmacies, and critical equipment storage, where environmental conditions directly impact care quality and energy usage. Even a network of a few dozens of strategically placed sensors can provide valuable insights to begin a hospital's innovation journey. Furthermore, empowering patients with direct control over their immediate environment, for example, through a bedside entertainment and communication terminal that manages lighting, window shades, temperature, and potentially ventilation, enhances well-being and alleviates staff workload. Infopoints and digital registration terminals reduce waiting times while improving patient experience, especially if pre-registration from home is already possible.

Stage 2: Automated Hospital
Building on a sensor foundation, the next stage involves creating automated responses to the data being collected. At this level, the building management systems begin to communicate with each other through software platforms that connect between different systems.

For example, when occupancy sensors detect an empty room, automated systems adjust lighting, temperature, and ventilation accordingly. Simple scheduling automation can reduce energy consumption significantly while maintaining optimal conditions when spaces are in use. Real-time location services (RTLS) [12] can track the availability of clean beds within a pre-defined area; upon the removal of a bed from this area for patient use, a logistics request for a replacement can be automatically initiated.

This stage also involves implementing basic predictive maintenance alerts for critical infrastructure to prevent failures before they impact operations.

Stage 3: Smart Hospital
Once the building infrastructure is automated, the necessary foundations are in place to become a smart hospital. Success hinges on one critical factor: interoperability. The ability to connect devices means that all components can meaningfully exchange and interpret data through an open protocol.

For instance, the efficiency of hospital logistics utilizing autonomously guided vehicles (AGVs) is significantly enhanced when logistics requests are automatically generated from the hospital information system's surgery schedule. Furthermore, AGVs can leverage real-time location system (RTLS) IoT sensors for navigation, integrate with the building management system for elevator control, and optimize charging based on surplus solar power and remaining transportation capacity, all orchestrated by a central fleet and charging management system. Ultimately, smart hospitals harness this integrated data from building infrastructure to generate predictive and prescriptive insights, thereby optimizing overall hospital operations and facility management.

Stage 4: Autonomous Hospital
The next phase of the journey is one where hospitals evolve into autonomous facilities, driven by real-time insights from connected, aggregated data and robust Industrial AI. While this remains a forward-looking aspiration rather than current reality, it represents the ultimate destination on the digital transformation roadmap. Some aspects of this vision are already a reality with AI-powered insights that help buildings adapt autonomously to changes in use or provide predictive maintenance recommendations to maximize uptime and minimize disruption to care. Moreover, the integration of functional Digital Twins, built upon Building Information

Modeling (BIM) data, can establish a "Lifecycle Twin." Such a twin not only facilitates process simulations for proactive planning but also supports continuous adaptation of operational processes.

9.2.2 A Helping Hand for Financing and Implementation

While the benefits of becoming a smart hospital are clear, the financial investment required can seem daunting innovative financing models (e.g., outcome-based financing or digital infrastructure leasing) represent crucial enablers for smart hospital implementation. Unlike traditional capital funding models, smart healthcare finance provides flexible options that align with individual digital maturity journeys, helping institutions better manage resources, reduce costs, embrace efficiency, and ultimately create a healthier future for all.

The challenges of transformation extend beyond finance. Investing in smart building technology can be a complex undertaking if in-house digitalization expertise, to make the right decisions for a hospital, isn't available. With more than 70% of digital transformation initiatives falling short on their objectives [13], it's essential to work with experienced partners who will be a compass, ensuring the hospital always heads in the right direction on its digitalization journey.

The future of hospitals is undoubtedly digital, and a digital transformation journey is needed to meet the complex challenges in healthcare. This journey becomes less daunting when approached collaboratively, holistically, and in manageable steps, understanding that meaningful transformation takes time.

9.3 Business Case and Return of Investment

The business case for smart hospital adoption is compelling. It was demonstrated that digital health solutions can deliver a return on investment within one year for new buildings and within two years for retrofitted facilities [14]. Key drivers include energy savings from smart lighting and HVAC systems, space optimization through data-driven planning, and workflow efficiency enabled by automation. These improvements not only reduce costs but also enhance revenue potential by increasing patient throughput and minimizing administrative overhead. Quantitative benefits include reduced CO_2 emissions [15], increased bed capacity, and improved compliance with hygiene protocols.

Real-world implementations underscore the effectiveness of this supplier-led approach. At Sint Maarten Hospital in Belgium [16], a single integrated building management system coordinates power, security, and environmental controls, creating a responsive and resilient care environment. At Ankara City Hospital in Türkiye [17], one of the largest hospital campuses globally, one command center manages over 800,000 data points across 22 subsystems, ensuring operational continuity and safety at scale. Kantonsspital Baden [18], a brand-new hospital in Switzerland, became the country's smartest hospital when it opened in 2025. Industry players worked in partnership with the hospital's development team to create a unique offer which uses digital tools and services to build an IoT platform in which solutions to specific challenges can be tailored, added, and scaled as they arise. Together they have delivered a customized IoT smart hospital platform which uses 2000 asset tags and 7000 IoT sensors to help patients and staff find their way around the hospital using app-based navigation, and a real-time location service to keep track of critical assets, such as beds and wheelchairs [19, 20].

9.4 Conclusion

These examples illustrate how digital transformation, when guided by a strategic framework and executed in partnership with experienced suppliers, can fundamentally reshape hospital operations. By aligning infrastructure modernization with clinical and operational goals, hospitals can navigate current challenges while positioning themselves for future success.

The adoption of digital health solutions in hospital settings requires more than technology. It demands a comprehensive framework that addresses complexity, fosters collaboration, and delivers measurable outcomes. By aligning infrastructure modernization with strategic goals, hospitals can navigate the challenges of today while preparing for the demands of tomorrow.

References

1. United Nations. Shifting demographics. United Nations; 2020. https://www.un.org/en/un75/shifting-demographics. Accessed 09 Oct 2025.
2. von Siemens B, Herrero-Yraola A. The Energy Paradox in healthcare: How to Balance Innovation with Sustainability. World Economic Forum, Jan. 20, 2025. https://www.weforum.org/stories/2025/01/the-energy-paradox-in-healthcare-how-to-balance-innovation-with-sustainability/
3. WHO. Health Workforce. www.who.int. 2021. https://www.who.int/health-topics/health-workforce. Accessed 09 Oct 2025.
4. Serbanati LD. Health digital state and smart EHR systems. Inform Med Unlock. 2020;21:100494. https://doi.org/10.1016/j.imu.2020.100494.
5. Berwick DM, Nolan TW, Whittington J. The triple aim: care, health, and cost. Health affairs (Project Hope). 2008;27(3):759–69. https://doi.org/10.1377/hlthaff.27.3.759.
6. Kasrineh M, Soodejani M. Smart hospitals worldwide: a systematic review. Physiol Pharmacol. 2023;27(3) https://doi.org/10.52547/phypha.27.3.2.
7. Ilyashenko O, Ilin I, Kurapeev D. Smart hospital concept and its implementation capabilities based on the incentive extension. SHS Web Conf. 2018;44:00040. https://doi.org/10.1051/shsconf/20184400040.
8. Pan American Health Organization (PAHO). Smart Hospitals Initiative - PAHO/WHO | Pan American Health Organization. www.paho.org. https://www.paho.org/en/smarthospitals. Accessed 10 Oct 2025.
9. Siemens AG. The Future of Care - the Smart Hospital Digital Transformation. Siemens Switzerland Ltd; 2023 [Online]. Available: https://assets.new.siemens.com/siemens/assets/api/uuid:d743a28c-95dd-46f8-a7e4-17817999e0f3/WP-Smart-hospitals-WHY-en_original.pdf. Accessed 10 Oct 2025.

10. WHO Foundation. Five fast facts on healthcare's climate footprint. www.who.foundation. 2024. https://wwwwhofoundation/post/five-fast-facts-on-healthcares-climate-footprint. Accessed 09 Oct 2025.
11. Greene-Dewasmes G, Tladi T. AI's Energy dilemma: challenges, opportunities, and a path forward. World Economic Forum, Jan. 21, 2025. https://www.weforum.org/stories/2025/01/ai-energy-dilemma-challenges-opportunities-and-path-forward/. Accessed 10 Oct 2025.
12. Frost & Sullivan, RTLS essential for location awareness—the key to solving business problems. Frost & Sullivan, Sep. 11, 2018. https://www.frost.com/growth-opportunity-news/rtls-essential-for-location-awareness-the-key-to-solving-business-problems/. Accessed 09 Oct 2025.
13. BCG. Flipping the Odds of Digital Transformation Success. 2020 [Online]. Available: https://web-assets.bcg.com/c7/20/907821344bbb8ade98cbe10fc2b8/bcg-flipping-the-odds-of-digital-transformation-success-oct-2020.pdf. Accessed 10 Oct 2025.
14. Siemens AG. Siemens Xcelerator Whitepaper: safeguard your smart hospital digital transformation. siemenscom. Global Website. 2024. https://xcelerator.siemens.com/global/en/industries/healthcare/documents-resources/siemens-xcelerator-whitepaper-smart-hospital-digital-transformation.html. Accessed 09 Oct 2025.
15. Pichler P-P, Jaccard IS, Weisz U, Weisz H. International comparison of health care carbon footprints. Environ Res Lett. 2019;14(6):064004. https://doi.org/10.1088/1748-9326/ab19e1.
16. Siemens AG. Sint-Maarten Hospital, Belgium. siemens.com Global Website. 2025. https://www.siemens.com/global/en/products/buildings/references/sint-maarten-hospital.html. Accessed 09 Oct 2025.
17. Siemens AG. Ankara City Hospital, Türkiye. siemens.com Global Website. 2025. https://www.siemens.com/global/en/products/buildings/references/smart-building-management-system-ankara-city-hospital.html. Accessed 09 Oct 2025.
18. Siemens AG. Ein Smart Hospital Mit 600 Jahren Tradition. Siemens. 2025. https://www.siemens.com/de/de/produkte/gebaeudetechnik/referenzen/kantonsspital-baden.html. Accessed 09 Oct 2025.
19. Siemens Schweiz. Siemens IoT-Technologie macht Kantonsspital Baden zu einem der intelligentesten Krankenhäuser der Schweiz | Presse | Siemens. Siemenscom. 2024. https://press.siemens.com/ch/de/pressemitteilung/siemens-iot-technologie-macht-kantonsspital-baden-zu-einem-der-intelligentesten. Accessed 09 Oct 2025.
20. Baden K. Willkommen im Spital der Zukunft. ksb - Das Gesundheitsmagazin für den Kanton Aargau, no. 4, 2024 [Online]. Available: https://www.kantonsspitalbaden.ch/documents/2024-11/ksb-4-24-aargau-sprint.pdf. Accessed 09 Oct 2025.

Part IV

AI and Digital Transformation in Ambulatory Care

AI Applications in Ambulatory Medical Practice: Lessons from Digital Transformation

10

Kerstin Dornauer

10.1 AI-Supported Diagnostics in Outpatient Care

In medical practices, classic heuristic questions are frequently observed, which are characteristic in their recurrence in everyday working life. Heuristics are defined as cognitive strategies that enable quick decisions to be made or problems to be solved in uncertain or complex situations. This is particularly relevant in the context of medical diagnoses. The likelihood that the practitioner will come up with a particular problem-solving strategy is influenced by the internal cognitive availability of the diagnosis and by distorted perceptions of patients due to their external circumstances. Doctors tend to rely on a specific solution approach when making a diagnosis and tend to place more trust in the diagnoses of their superiors than in their own beliefs [1]. Stress, lack of time, fatigue, and overload further exacerbate the problems and thus make it difficult to systematically collate the diagnostic data collected. AI can help address the challenges described above in diagnostics and treatment decisions by analyzing all available data on a treated person and, if necessary, comparing it with scientific literature [2]. It offers a "second opinion," questions clinical decisions, or points out when important information or connections may not have been taken into account. Algorithms that aim to support decision-making in the areas of diagnosis and therapy are referred to as clinical decision support systems [3].

Imaging techniques play an essential role in medical diagnostics in almost all specialist areas. The higher flow rate of diagnostics with the same staffing levels during the same period currently poses a structural challenge for the field of radiology both in clinical and private practice settings. Added to this is the requirement for precise diagnosis of particularly small abnormalities and the exact estimation of three-dimensional extensions with increasing image quality. This is where image analysis software tools come in, which use AI to support the evaluation of X-ray,

K. Dornauer (✉)
Dr. Dornauer & Colleagues, Zirndorf, Germany

S. Scholz et al. (eds.), *Advancements in Digital Health and Care*,
https://doi.org/10.1007/978-3-032-16837-5_10

CT, and MRI images. Despite the ongoing digital transformation in Germany and increasing digitalization in healthcare, the development of trustworthy AI in the field of medical imaging often proves difficult, as only small amounts of data (little data) are available, especially in the case of rare diseases. For the development and evaluation of AI models, extensive amounts of data (big data) are essential to ensure high precision and reliability of AI decisions [4].

FAST (feedback-guided automation of sub-tasks), a project run by the Fraunhofer Institute, has the aim of finding a solution to these problems, to automate decisions, and therefore processes, using an AI component. FAST essentially consists of two components: an AI component making predictions about the captured images, and a second component quantifying the reliability of these predictions and thus deciding which data can be processed automatically. The central question is how an AI model can be trained to enable reliable predictions even when only limited training data is available. To this end, FAST introduces the concept of "subproblems." A subproblem is defined by the training data that the system can learn early on and by a significantly smaller number of examples than would be required for the overall problem [5].

As part of the project "Highly Reliable QC-Based Artificial Intelligence for Medical Diagnosis Tasks," which is being carried out in collaboration with the Medical Centre of Ludwig Maximilian University in Munich, Fraunhofer IKS is gaining to optimize medical diagnosis through the use of hybrid quantum computing-based machine learning models. The hybrid approach, which combines quantum technology and classical methods, offers the advantage that a NISQ (Noisy Intermediate-Scale Quantum) quantum computer can be used for this purpose [6]. The current quantum computing approaches have the potential to bring about significant progress in the field of AI-supported diagnostic processes. Therefore, quantum computing has the potential to train AI more efficiently in medical diagnostics. This enables more accurate diagnoses, even when data are limited [6].

Another area of application for AI-supported diagnostics is dermatology due to skin cancer diagnosis. Melanoma is responsible for most skin cancer-related deaths worldwide. However, distinguishing between early-stage melanoma and other skin tumors proves difficult. Recent advances in AI-based diagnostic support systems have the potential to help dermatologists diagnose melanoma and birthmarks more accurately by presenting them with digitized images of suspicious lesions. Doctors strive to understand the characteristics that determine the results of AI systems, as they ultimately bear primary responsibility for the diagnosis. Judgments made in relation to AI-based systems must be traceable with regard to the selection parameters applied. The objective was therefore to design a support system that is tailored to the perspective of dermatologists in the context of melanoma diagnosis and explains their decision-making process. The development of explainable AI (XAI) aimed to strengthen user confidence in AI support. XAI is the ability of AI systems to provide clear and understandable explanations for their actions and decisions [7–9]. Its central goal is to make the behavior of these systems understandable to humans by elucidating the underlying mechanisms of their decision-making processes. The AI is capable of providing dermatologically plausible explanations, as it refers to the characteristics of specific, individual zones of the lesion. A three-phase study examined the impact on diagnostic accuracy, diagnostic certainty, and dermatologists' confidence in the explanatory system. Over a hundred dermatologists from 33 different countries participated in the randomized study. The doctors diagnosed a test panel of digitized images of various lesions three times—based on their experience alone, with the support of a conventional AI system and with the XAI. Previous studies have already documented that the use of an AI system increases diagnostic accuracy in the detection of melanoma. While AI systems improved melanoma detection accuracy, adding XAI primarily enhanced clinicians' confidence rather than diagnostic accuracy. The use of AI technology also improved dermatologists' confidence in their own decisions, with the increase being even more pronounced when using the XAI system. It was found that the confidence of physicians in their own diagnoses was highly dependent on the consistency of their decision criteria with those listed by the XAI. The results demonstrate that XAI can optimize the diagnostic confidence of clinicians and has the potential to increase the acceptance of AI methods among physicians. According to the European General Data Protection Regulation, the interpretation of decisions relevant to the end user that are based on algorithms is mandatory. This is significant for the successful use of AI-based software in dermatology [10, 11].

Although AI is becoming increasingly widespread, many of these systems function in ways that are disadvantageous to users. In the complex world of AI systems, even the providers of these systems are often unable to adequately interpret and understand the decisions and results of the systems they have developed. This phenomenon is known as the "black box" effect [12–14].

10.2 Optimizing Workflows and Practice Management with AI

The use of AI has the potential to support a wide range of work processes in medical practices [15]. It should be noted that this technology does not replace the expertise of a medical professional or human contact. Rather, it helps to make routine and analytical tasks more efficient. As a result, more time is available for patient care. This idea becomes even more striking considering, that, in average, over 50% of the time spent by established colleagues is taken with administrative tasks. The following areas are particularly relevant in this context:

10.2.1 Patient Communication and Appointment Management

AI-supported chat or telephone assistants answer frequently asked questions, take prescription requests, and can guide patients to some available appointments. They are reachable around the clock and can handle simple requests independently. Currently, AI benefits practices mainly in easily delegated organizational tasks. However, full automation of complex practice planning is not yet feasible due to inconsistent workflows. This circumstance is due to the inconsistency of the organizational structures, which consequently cannot be reliably mapped. Another part of AI-optimized practice management is an online reception which offers patients questionnaires download. Patients can fill out their medical history online at home before they enter the office physically. AI processes the uploaded data and integrates it into the practice software for more effectivity.

10.2.2 Scheduling and Reminding

AI efficiently assigns appointments, takes into account capacity utilization, no-show forecasts, and reminds patients of follow-up appointments in good time. There is the option of sending approved treatment and cost plans to both, patients and the treating practice, using AI and messenger services. This has the advantage of avoiding time-consuming search processes and high administrative costs, which are common in larger practices. Patients are simultaneously notified via a messaging service that their desired treatment can begin and are asked to make an appointment therefore. AI systems are capable of analyzing findings and laboratory values, extracting essential information and assisting with correct coding and billing. Automated follow-up reminders serve as a tool for increasing compliance by informing patients about checkups, vaccinations, and recall intervals. In everyday practice, automated patient recall helps to reduce the administrative burden on the practice. Patients are identified using an algorithm that filters out those patients who are due for their next preventive checkup and then contacts them.

10.2.3 Organization Management, Resources, Costs

In the organizational area of a practice, AI can help to increase the efficiency of resource allocation. By automating routinc tasks and prioritizing tasks according to their availability, AI can help tailor the use of staff and premises to specific needs. It is evident that speech-processing programs and AI assistants make a significant contribution to the optimization of documentation processes. They support the transcription of patient consultations and enable the automated transfer of relevant content to electronic patient records.

In the area of practice organization, AI-based systems can identify material shortages and initiate automated, timely reordering. This has the advantage of not only avoiding a high administrative burden but also maintaining a cost- and benefit-optimized warehouse that always keeps an eye on demand. Time-consuming inventories are therefore no longer necessary.

The optimization of work processes in medical practices through the use of AI is particularly evident in the automation of routine tasks, accelerated access to information, and support in diagnostics and therapy. The software relieves staff of the burden of scheduling appointments, documentation, coding and patient communication. At the same time, data protection, quality control, and medical responsibility are essential elements of the medical profession. AI systems generate suggestions and offer support, particularly in the administrative area. This leads to significant time savings, allowing doctors to spend more time treating their patients.

10.2.4 AI in Modern Dental Practices

Intraoral scanners have been an established part of dentistry for many years now, replacing traditional methods of taking impressions of teeth using impression material. AI-supported intraoral scanners are characterized by their combination of high-resolution optical capture and intelligent algorithms. These systems go beyond mere "digital impressions" and offer significant advantages for the treatment team and patients. Modern scanners are user-friendly, wireless and can be easily integrated into existing workflows. Thanks to the AI used, the scanner easily returns to its original task even after interruptions in recording or replacing the battery. Digital recording replaces manual mixing of impression material and plaster models. Data can be sent directly to the dental laboratory, significantly reducing production times for restorations. AI-based CAD/CAM (computer-aided design/computer-aided manufacturing) software recognizes anatomical structures and automatically leads to creating restorations or drilling templates. This enables fast design and production processes, so that, for example, a complete "smile design" can be discussed with the patient within an hour. Intraoral scanners generate a precise 3D model in a fraction of a second, which AI analyzes in real time and filters out even the smallest deviations. This ensures excellent precision of the images even in areas that are difficult to access. From the patient's point of view, the main advantage is the noninvasive generation of image data, which does not pose any challenges for them, because there are no uncomfortable impression trays or gagging, which anxious patients in particular find reassuring. Patients immediately see a 3D model of their teeth, realistic visualizations, and treatment simulations, which facilitate decision-making and increase confidence.

The use of AI-based intraoral scanners streamlines the workflow, as these devices automatically process data, reduce sources of error, and enable rapid transfer to digital manufacturing systems. Early detection of caries and automatic planning contribute to improving diagnostic accuracy and the quality of dental prostheses. For patients, the examinations offer advantages in terms of comfort, speed, and clear visualizations. In addition, patient anxiety is reduced and cooperation with the treatment team is promoted.

In dental technology, CAD/CAM programs based on deep learning algorithms enable the automated recognition of structures and the generation of design proposals for crowns, bridges, and splints. In addition, the available algorithm technology allows morphological duplicates to be created. The acceleration of the dental prosthesis production process, increased patient satisfaction, and the reduction of manual errors on the part of dental technicians are significant advantages associated with the digital manufacturing process [16].

10.2.5 Cost-Benefit Analysis for Small- and Medium-Sized Practices

The economic viability of investments in AI for small- and medium-sized practices depends on the intended areas of application, the costs, and the resources of the practice. The following facts contribute to the benefit assessment:

Efficiency gains—One of the most important strengths of AI is the automation of routine tasks.
Greater diagnostic certainty and targeted treatment—AI algorithms analyze intraoral scans, X-ray, and CT images in real time; detect subtle patterns, and provide early indications of caries, periodontitis, or other anomalies.
Greater patient comfort and higher acceptance—Contactless digital impressions prevent gagging and breathing difficulties.
Increasing affordability—According to market observations, modern scanners are smaller, wireless, and significantly cheaper than they were just a few years ago.
Relieving staff in times of skilled worker shortages—Automated assistance systems can handle the flood of calls per day at the practice and relieve the existing staff, leaving more time for patient care.

AI systems involve initial acquisition and licensing costs as well as training for the team [17].

10.2.6 Evaluation for Small- and Medium-Sized Practices

In short term, practices with limited staff will benefit particularly from telephone assistants, automated appointment scheduling, and digital documentation. The implementation of these applications involves low costs and results in a rapid, noticeable reduction in workload and an improvement in quality.

It can be assumed that an AI-supported intraoral scanner will have a significant impact on treatment quality in the medium term and will lead to an increase in revenue. The purchase involves higher costs, but leads to time savings once the workflow within the practice has been optimized.

In the long term, the digitalization of the practice promises a competitive advantage: efficiency, modern treatment, and positive patient experiences strengthen the reputation and increase utilization.

For a large number of small- and medium-sized dental practices, investing in AI will prove profitable, provided that it is designed to meet their needs and that staff receive adequate training. The benefits are particularly evident in the form of time savings, optimized diagnostics, and increased patient satisfaction.

10.3 Interoperability and Data Integration in Ambulatory Settings

The digital transformation of a medical practice involves more than just implementing new devices. Rather, it requires the seamless integration of practice management, diagnostics, and laboratory services. In practical application, three significant barriers to integration become apparent:

10.3.1 Practice Management

The current software landscape is highly fragmented and characterized by poor interoperability. A significant number of digital applications, such as online appointment booking, telemedicine, and e-prescription systems, are usually implemented separately from the primary practice software, as interfaces are often not integrated. Although proprietary interfaces exist for individual applications, duplicate data entry or manual transfer of to-dos into the practice software is usually the norm. Appointments booked via an online reception desk often have to be entered manually into the main calendar. Manual entry of e-prescriptions and electronic certificates of incapacity for work (eAU) is also frequently required. There is no universally applicable set of rules that clearly defines interoperability between the various IT solutions used in medical practices. In the outpatient sector, there are currently no legally prescribed interfaces such as those specified by the ISiK standards for hospitals.

The widespread opening up of practice software as a game changer:

Some providers apparently intend to open up their systems to other applications via an FHIR-based standard interface [18].

Until these interfaces are implemented and certified across the board, practices will continue to be forced to work with proprietary solutions and manual processes.

The following must be taken into account with regard to personnel and legal requirements:

In addition to technical interfaces, the digital competence of personnel poses a significant challenge. In many cases, there is a lack of training measures that enable the efficient use of new systems.

Furthermore, the applicable data protection and telematics requirements must be taken into account, such as gematik approval of components.

10.3.2 Medical Imaging

Integrating medical technology requires modern practice management solutions that offer interfaces for connecting ultrasound, endoscopy, and digital X-ray systems. In practical application, however, technical integration of the devices, configuration of data transfers, and training of staff are necessary. This requires a great deal of effort and specific IT expertise.

With regard to data formats and system selection, the following should be noted:

In dentistry, it is essential that digital scanners and imaging systems are compatible with the software used in the laboratory. The appropriate selection of software and ensuring system compatibility, particularly in the context of data exchange between the practice and the laboratory or between the scanner and in-house production, is therefore of significant importance for a smooth digital process.

Open versus closed systems:

Open imaging systems export standard formats such as STL (Standard Triangle Language) or DICOM (Digital Imaging and Communications in Medicine), enabling further processing in third-party software. However, it should be noted that some manufacturers encode their "open" files so that they only work with their own software.

Closed systems work well internally, but tie the practice to one provider and make it harder to integrate with external programs.

10.3.3 (Dental) Laboratory Connection

The harmonization of interfaces is of essential importance. In the context of transferring digital impressions or laboratory orders in dental offices, it is essential that the relevant file (e.g., in STL format) can be imported directly into the laboratory's CAD software. Subsequently, after the design has been completed, a corresponding transfer file is transferred to the CAM software. To ensure optimal results, the harmonization of interfaces is of crucial importance. This means that the data from the intraoral scanner must be compatible with the CAD software in the laboratory. In traditional medical practices, the interfaces of the practice management software should be compatible with all external data that is to be imported. Under optimal conditions, the data can then be imported directly into the patient file and stored there in a personalized manner.

10.3.4 ePA—Opportunities and Risks

The electronic patient record (ePA) is a central component of the German healthcare system's digitalization strategy. Like a digital health folder, it is intended to make findings, doctor's letters, X-ray images, and medication plans available in one place. For private practices, this presents opportunities, but also risks in terms of data integration and interoperability.

Advantages for interoperability and practice workflow:

The centralization of information and the avoidance of duplicate examinations are key objectives pursued by the ePA. With the consent of the insured, doctors have the opportunity to view all relevant documents. This eliminates the need for duplicate examinations and makes the exchange of treatment data on paper or by fax superfluous.

The flow of information in the context of referrals and emergencies has been optimized. In the event of a referral to a specialist, the specialist is able to view the existing documents in the ePA and add their own report.

In an emergency, important information is immediately available, which increases patient safety.

According to the Federal Ministry of Health, the ePA will be expanded to include a digital medication plan starting in 2025. This measure aims to improve the detection of drug interactions and facilitate the management of electronic prescriptions.

The resulting time savings and patient involvement are significant advantages. Patients no longer have to collect paper files and have access to their health data at any time. In addition, they can obtain second opinions more easily and change doctors more simply. For medical practices, this means less effort in taking medical histories and more efficient documentation.

10.3.5 Risks and Challenges

Data security and technical infrastructure—Data protection experts point out that the central storage of sensitive health data is an attractive target for attacks. In 2024, the Chaos Computer Club generated a significant number of access keys that can be traced back to security vulnerabilities. Although the data in the telematics infrastructure is encrypted and only approved file formats are used, there is still a residual risk of hacking or misuse. Fragmentation and a lack of standardization pose significant challenges. The Federation of German Consumer Organisations criticizes the fact that each of the 95 health insurance companies offers its own ePA app. This results in high resource expenditure and information deficits for consumers. Numerous digital applications are used in doctors' offices that are operated separately from the practice software. This means that information from online reception, telemedicine, or eAU must be transferred manually. As long as no binding, standardized interfaces are established, the aspects of interoperability and continuous workflow remain a challenge. There are technical and organizational obstacles that can interfere with smooth access to the ePA. For example, a stable internet connection is required to access the electronic patient record. In addition, up-to-date practice software is crucial to ensure data integrity and security. It should be noted that system failures or a slower internet connection can make access difficult. For doctors, the ePA offers the possibility of optimized networking. The electronic sharing of findings, X-ray images, and medication plans between different medical disciplines makes it possible to avoid duplicate examinations and improve patient care. This results in a significant improvement in the quality of treatment and the exchange of information. At the same time, practices are confronted with technical and organizational challenges: the absence of standards for connecting practice administration, imaging, and laboratories complicates integration and data protection. Successful use of the ePA requires investment in a secure IT infrastructure, training for the practice team and a willingness to establish new processes.

10.4 Lessons Learned

Experience gained in the first few years of using AI systems shows that their potential is considered to be enormous, but that a number of prerequisites and framework conditions are necessary for successful implementation. Several lessons can be learned from the steps taken so far [19]:

The potential has been recognized, but its use is still selective. A Bitkom survey conducted in May 2025 among more than 600 doctors shows that AI is already being used in one in seven practices. Nearly, 12% of respondents use it to support diagnoses and 8% in practice management.

A recent study has shown that 78% of doctors consider AI to be a significant opportunity and are calling for targeted promotion.

However, the available usage figures suggest that widespread use in the outpatient sector is still in its infancy [20].

Interoperability and data integration are identified as key challenges. In many practices, digital services (online reception, eAU, telemedicine) are currently still operated separately from the practice software, which requires manual transfers.

Although open standards such as FHIR are the subject of discussion, they are still in the development phase in the outpatient sector.

The lack of interfaces is a significant factor limiting the benefits of AI. In order to ensure efficient linking of data from imaging, administrative software, and laboratories, it is necessary to establish interoperable systems and binding interfaces.

The quality of the data is crucial to the quality of the AI. Fraunhofer IKS emphasizes that the data set is the most time-consuming aspect of an AI project. Small data sets, multimedia data, and distributed data requiring protection require special approaches such as federated learning. Incorrect or incomplete data can cause uncertainties and bias in the models. An important lesson is therefore that practices must structure their data collection and ensure data quality before AI algorithms can be used effectively. The present Bitkom study shows that although 68% of doctors are generally open to electronic patient records, 77% feel insufficiently prepared for their use. This can be attributed to a lack of digital competence and training among staff. To realize AI's potential, training and workflow redesign should precede or accompany implementation rather than follow it. This usually does not lead to a reduction in workload, but rather to an increase in effort. The integration of AI into the workflow is therefore essential. Staff must be able to both understand and operate the systems. Ensuring data security and the legal framework are key aspects.

Security breaches, such as those that have occurred with electronic patient records, highlight the importance of robust protective measures. The future implementation of the EU AI Act and national data protection rules will have a significant impact on the success of the digital transformation.

References

1. Elstein AS. Evidence base of clinical diagnosis: clinical problem solving and diagnostic decision making: selective review of the cognitive literature. BMJ. 2002;324(7339):729–32.
2. Maleki Varnosfaderani S, Forouzanfar M. The role of AI in hospitals and clinics: transforming healthcare in the 21st century. Bioengineering. 2024;11(4):337.
3. Tschochohei M, Adams LC, Bressem KK, Lammert J. KI-gestützte klinische Entscheidungsunterstützungssysteme: Herausforderungen und Potenziale. Bundesgesundheitsbl. 2025;68(8):872–9.
4. Khalifa M, Albadawy M. AI in diagnostic imaging: revolutionising accuracy and efficiency. Comput Methods Programs Biomed Update. 2024;5:100146.
5. Wehinger L. FAST: Wie weniger Daten zu frühzeitiger und zuverlässiger Automatisierung durch KI führen. 2023. Available from: https://safe-intelligence.fraunhofer.de/artikel/visuelle-inspektion-zuverlaessige-automatisierung-durch-fast.
6. Lorenz JM. BayQS: Bayerisches Kompetenzzentrum quanten security und data science. Available from: https://www.iks.fraunhofer.de/de/projekte/bayqs-quanten-security-data-science.html#medizin.
7. Golden G, Popescu C, Israel S, Perlman K, Armstrong C, Fratila R, et al. Applying artificial intelligence to clinical decision support in mental health: what have we learned? Health Policy Technol. 2024;13(2):100844.
8. Chanda T, Hauser K, Hobelsberger S, Bucher TC, Garcia CN, Wies C, et al. Dermatologist-like explainable AI enhances trust and confidence in diagnosing melanoma. Nat Commun. 2024;15(1):524.
9. Chanda T, Haggenmueller S, Bucher TC, Holland-Letz T, Kittler H, Tschandl P, et al. Dermatologist-like explainable AI enhances melanoma diagnosis accuracy: eye-tracking study. Nat Commun. 2025;16(1):4739.
10. Manole I, Second Dermatology Department, Colentina Clinical Hospital, Bucharest, Romania, Second Dermatology Discipline, "Carol Davila" University of Medicine and Pharmacy, Bucharest, Romania. Integrating Artificial Intelligence in dermatology: progress, challenges and perspectives. Ro Med J 2024;71(2):183–191.
11. Behara K, Bhero E, Agee JT. AI in dermatology: a comprehensive review into skin cancer detection. PeerJ Comput Sci. 2024;10:e2530.
12. Kosinski M. What is black box AI? 2024. Available from: https://www.ibm.com/think/topics/black-box-ai.
13. Marcus E, Teuwen J. Artificial intelligence and explanation: how, why, and when to explain black boxes. Eur J Radiol. 2024;173:111393.
14. Xu H, Shuttleworth KMJ. Medical artificial intelligence and the black box problem: a view based on the ethical principle of "do no harm". Intell Med. 2024;4(1):52–7.
15. Rybakov A. How to ensure healthcare efficiency with the power of AI workflow automation. 2025. Available from: https://spsoft.com/tech-insights/ai-workflow-automation-for-healthcare/.
16. Gomez Rossi J, Rojas-Perilla N, Krois J, Schwendicke F. Cost-effectiveness of artificial intelligence as a decision-support system applied to the detection and grading of melanoma, dental caries, and diabetic retinopathy. JAMA Netw Open. 2022;5(3):e220269.
17. El Arab RA, Al Moosa OA. Systematic review of cost effectiveness and budget impact of artificial intelligence in healthcare. NPJ Digit Med. 2025;8(1):548.

18. Halilaj M, Vasil S, Kosta A, Lili I. Interoperability within healthcare systems through FHIR. Artif Intell Cloud Integ IJEATS. 2025;13(1):22–8.
19. Krishna A, Friend D, Gohad N, Reddy P. The coming evolution of healthcare AI toward a modular architecture. 2025. Available from: https://www.mckinsey.com/industries/healthcare/our-insights/the-coming-evolution-of-healthcare-ai-toward-a-modular-architecture.
20. Bitkom e.V. KI in fast jeder siebten Praxis und vielen Kliniken im Einsatz. 2025. Available from: https://www.bitkom.org/Presse/Presseinformation/KI-in-Praxis-und-Kliniken-im-Einsatz.

Part V

Patient-Centered Perspectives in the Digital Health Ecosystem

Patient-Centric Approaches to Digital Health: Payer Evaluation on the Utilization and Development of Digital Health

11

Ute Irene Wiedemann

11.1 Introduction

Digital transformation has become a defining feature of modern health systems. The integration of mobile health technologies, artificial intelligence, and patient-driven digital tools into care processes has created both opportunities and challenges for health policy. At the center of this transformation lies the question of how digital health applications can strengthen patient autonomy, improve access to care, and deliver measurable outcomes under the constraints of solidarity-based health financing [1, 2]. Germany was the first country worldwide to systematically include digital health applications (World Health Organization 2021, Digitale Gesundheitsanwendungen, DiGA) in statutory health insurance coverage. Since the adoption of the Digitale-Versorgung-Gesetz (DVG) in 2019, insured persons have been legally entitled to reimbursement of listed DiGA, creating a unique framework for innovation and patient empowerment [3]. The German DiGA model has thus become a reference point for international health systems, inspiring similar approaches in the countries France and Belgium [9, 10]. This chapter examines patient-centric approaches to digital health from the perspective of payers, with a specific focus on the development and utilization of DiGA. Section 11.2 outlines the policy frameworks that govern access and reimbursement, while Sect. 11.3 analyzes strategic approaches to digital transformation in healthcare. Section 11.4 traces the evolution of DiGA from pilot projects to national infrastructure, and Section 11.5 explores utilization patterns and associated challenges. Finally, Section 11.6 critically examines reimbursement mechanisms and payer perspectives, situating the German model in comparison with other countries including the United Kingdom, the United States, and European initiatives. By synthesizing policy, strategic, and financial perspectives, this chapter seeks to highlight both the potential and the

U. I. Wiedemann (✉)
DAK-Gesundheit, Mitglied des Vorstandes, Hamburg, Germany
e-mail: ute.wiedemann@dak.de

S. Scholz et al. (eds.), *Advancements in Digital Health and Care*,
https://doi.org/10.1007/978-3-032-16837-5_11

limitations of digital health reimbursement models. It emphasizes that the sustainable integration of digital therapeutics depends on reducing bureaucratic barriers, aligning incentives across stakeholders, and embedding outcome-based approaches into broader value-based healthcare strategies [6–8].

11.2 Policy Frameworks

The development and implementation of policy frameworks for digital health applications illustrate how health systems balance patient rights, regulatory oversight, and payer sustainability in the context of rapidly evolving innovation. Germany is the first country worldwide to create a statutory entitlement for digital therapeutics, guaranteeing reimbursement within the health insurance system [1–3]. Other countries, such as France, Belgium, the United Kingdom, and the United States, have taken more selective or fragmented approaches. At the international level, the European Union has advanced initiatives such as the European Health Data Space (EHDS) and the Artificial Intelligence Act (AI Act), which provide a broader regulatory backdrop for national strategies [14, 15].

The Digitale-Versorgung-Gesetz (DVG, 2019) amended Social Code Book V (§ 33a SGB V) to grant insured persons a legal entitlement to reimbursement of digital health applications once listed in the Federal Institute for Drugs and Medical Devices (BfArM) directory [2, 3]. Manufacturers of CE-marked medical devices of risk class I or IIa can apply for the "DiGA Fast-Track," if they can demonstrate a positive healthcare effect, which may consist either of direct medical benefit or of patient-relevant improvements in care processes such as adherence or accessibility [2]. Provisional listing guarantees reimbursement for twelve months while manufacturers generate additional evidence, typically through randomized controlled trials or comparative studies. If evidence is sufficient, permanent listing follows; if not, the application is removed from the directory [2].

Reimbursement negotiations are carried out with the GKV-Spitzenverband, the National Association of Statutory Health Insurance Funds. During the first twelve months after listing, manufacturers may set their own prices. After this period, prices are negotiated and applied retrospectively. This mechanism ensures rapid access for patients but also exposes manufacturers to financial risks if repayment obligations exceed revenues. For payers, the retrospective correction provides budgetary security and prevents uncontrolled cost escalation [4].

The German framework must also be situated within the broader European regulatory environment. Through the European Health Data Space (EHDS, 2022), primary and secondary use of health data are standardized, fostering interoperability across member states [14]. The AI Act, adopted in 2024, introduces a risk-based classification of artificial intelligence in medical devices, including digital therapeutics, thereby shaping the criteria for compliance and patient safety [15]. Other European countries have developed frameworks inspired by but distinct from Germany. France introduced the PECAN procedure in 2023, which allows temporary reimbursement of digital medical devices for twelve months, conditional on evidence of clinical or organizational benefit assessed by the Haute Autorité de Santé (HAS) [9]. Belgium launched the mHealth Belgium pyramid in 2019, a three-level certification and reimbursement system that requires compliance with safety and interoperability standards before reimbursement eligibility is granted [10]. These models reflect a selective adaptation of the German pathway, applying stricter evidence requirements and more limited budgetary scope.

The United Kingdom has chosen a different solution. Instead of creating a statutory entitlement, the NHS has developed standards under the National Institute for Health and Care Excellence (NICE), which provide evidence frameworks for digital health technologies and guide procurement [11]. This centralized approach ensures quality and safety but limits patient choice, as only centrally approved applications are reimbursed.

In the United States, the Food and Drug Administration (FDA) provides regulatory clearance for digital health applications through its Digital Health Center of Excellence, but coverage decisions remain fragmented. Medicare reimburses only specific services such as remote patient monitoring, while private insurers selectively cover certain digital therapeutics [12, 13]. This results in unequal access and limited scalability, as FDA approval does not guarantee reimbursement.

To enable systematic comparison, Table 11.1 summarizes the key features of five major policy frameworks.

This comparison shows that Germany remains the only country with a statutory entitlement embedded in its social insurance system, guaranteeing universal access once a DiGA is listed. France and Belgium have adopted selective adaptations that provide temporary or conditional reimbursement. The United Kingdom emphasizes centralized quality assurance through NICE and NHS procurement, while the United States illustrates the limitations of a market-driven approach where regulatory approval does not translate into systematic reimbursement.

Patient-centric digital health requires that innovation align with patient's values and expectations, not only with clinical efficacy. This includes transparent communication about data use, consent processes adapted to different levels of health literacy, and safeguards against bias to protect vulnerable groups. Embedding these

Table 11.1 Key features of five major policy frameworks

Country	Policy framework	Coverage/reimbursement model
Germany	DVG (2019), DiGAV, DigiG (2024); § 33a & § 134 SGB V	Free pricing 12 months, then negotiated tariff; retrospective repayment; outcome-based ≥20% from 2026
France	PECAN procedure (2023)	Temporary reimbursement (12 months), permanent listing after benefit review
Belgium	mHealth Belgium pyramid (2019–)	3-level system: safety → interoperability → reimbursement eligibility
UK (NHS)	NICE Evidence Standards Framework; NHS Long Term Plan	Centralized NHS procurement; NHS Apps Library
USA	FDA Digital Health Center of Excellence; Medicare pi lots	No uniform framework; fragmented coverage (Medicare RPM, private insurers)

principles at policy level strengthens trust, supports informed decision-making, and facilitates sustained engagement with digital interventions [1, 6, 7].

Operationalizing patient-centricity further entails choice and control for patients, while preserving clinician-patient relationship, such as preferred communication channels, feedback intensity, and the degree of automation. Professional guidance from medical staff underscores the need for explainability and appropriate oversight so that digital tools complement, rather than replace, clinical judgment [8].

11.3 Strategic Approaches to Digital Transformation in Healthcare

Germany's strategic approach is anchored in the national Digital Health Strategy, which emphasizes patient-centered use of electronic health records (ePA), interoperability, and integration of digital therapeutics [16]. In 2025, all insured persons received an ePA by default, allowing DiGA use to be directly integrated into patient records. Health insurers have also piloted digital infrastructures, such as app-based verification processes for DiGA prescriptions [17]. These initiatives demonstrate efforts to streamline administration and improve efficiency, although evaluations show that code issuance still frequently exceeds the legal two-day target [4].

Stakeholder collaboration is essential for governance. In Germany, this includes the BfArM for directory listing [2], the GKV-Spitzenverband for reimbursement negotiation [4], and the Kassenärztliche Bundesvereinigung (KBV) for integrating DiGA prescriptions into the Einheitlicher Bewertungsmaßstab (EBM), the national reimbursement catalog [18].

Industry partnerships play an important role in supporting patient-centric digital transformation. Collaborations between health technology firms, payers, and research institutions facilitate the validation of applications under real-world conditions, thereby accelerating safe and effective integration into care pathways [19]. Such alliances also enable the co-creation of tools with patient groups, ensuring that user needs and preferences are embedded from the outset [19]. By combining regulatory initiatives with industry-driven innovation, these partnerships can reduce barriers to access and improve usability across diverse patient populations. Evidence from European validation frameworks illustrates that participatory models contribute to higher acceptance and sustained engagement, particularly when cultural and linguistic adaptation is prioritized [10, 11].

Internationally, the NHS emphasizes centralized curation of digital tools, with NICE providing the evidence standards [11]. This ensures safety and quality but limits patient choice and flexibility since reimbursement depends on NHS procurement. The United States illustrates a market-driven model. The FDA provides regulatory approval [12], but reimbursement decisions are left to Medicare, Medicaid, and private insurers [13]. Medicare has introduced reimbursement codes for remote patient monitoring and telehealth, while private insurers selectively cover digital therapeutics [13].

These strategic differences reflect national priorities: Germany emphasizes legal entitlement, the NHS focuses on centralized safety and quality, and the United States fosters innovation through pluralism but at the cost of inequities in access. The German case demonstrates how statutory frameworks can accelerate digital adoption, but also how bureaucracy and financial risks can constrain innovation. Ultimately, effective digital transformation depends on aligning patient rights, evidence standards, and financial sustainability across stakeholders.

11.4 The Evolution of DiGA: From Pilot Projects to National Infrastructure and Patient-Centered Outcomes Measures

The evolution of the development of digital health applications in Germany can be traced in three phases: early experimentation through pilots, the establishment of a legal framework via the Digitale-Versorgung-Gesetz (DVG), and the creation of a national infrastructure integrating digital therapeutics into broader care pathways.

In the initial phase, prior to 2019, digital health applications were predominantly introduced within the framework of selective contracts and research pilot projects. Health insurers occasionally financed digital solutions such as telemonitoring programs for diabetes or mental health apps within limited populations [20, 21]. These pilots generated valuable insights into feasibility and patient acceptance but lacked scalability, since each project depended on local arrangements or temporary research funding. Patients' access was therefore uneven and restricted to specific insurance schemes or regions.

The second phase began with the adoption of the DVG in 2019, marking the transition from fragmented experimentation to a regulated reimbursement pathway [3]. With the creation of the DiGA directory, digital therapeutics could for the first time be prescribed nationwide and reimbursed by all statutory health insurers. By late 2024, 59 DiGA were listed, spanning therapeutic areas such as mental health, metabolic disorders, musculoskeletal conditions, and sleep medicine [4]. This institutionalization provided clarity for patients and providers: every insured person obtained the same legal entitlement once a DiGA was listed. Unlike the earlier pilot logic, access no longer depended on local insurer initiatives but became part of the statutory benefits catalogue.

In the third phase, the DiGA pathway evolved into a national digital infrastructure. By the end of 2024, nearly one million activation codes had been issued [4]. Most of these were prescribed by physicians, underscoring the continued centrality of medical professionals in the diffusion of DiGA [4]. Usage patterns show that adoption has been strongest among women and in the 50–64 age group, whereas uptake among younger adults and men remains lower [4]. Integration into the electronic patient record (ePA) and electronic prescription (eRezept), mandated by the 2024 Digital Act, represents the next step toward interoperability with other health services and the foundation for outcome-based reimbursement [5].

The institutionalization of DiGA has transformed the market landscape for digital therapeutics. Whereas early pilots were dominated by small startups, the current system requires increased investment in evidence generation, compliance with data protection, and negotiation capacities [21]. Several providers have exited the market due to financial strain, most prominently Aidhere, which declared insolvency in 2023 [22]. Retrospective repayment obligations after tariff negotiations proved unsustainable for smaller firms. Currently, major technology and pharmaceutical firms have entered the DiGA market, reflecting an ongoing transition from innovation predominantly driven by startups to a model increasingly shaped by established corporations [4]. This mirrors patterns in the United States, where FDA-approved digital therapeutics initially pioneered the field but later faced bankruptcy, only for larger companies to expand into the space [12, 13].

Germany's DiGA model has also influenced international policy. France and Belgium adapted aspects through the PECAN procedure and mHealth pyramid, respectively [9, 10]. The NHS has drawn on German experiences in shaping its standards and evidence requirements through the NICE framework [11]. The OECD has explicitly highlighted DiGA as a benchmark for integrating digital therapeutics into health technology assessment processes [19]. In the United States, selective reimbursement pilots by Medicare and private insurers indicate a growing interest in outcome-based models [13].

Beyond reimbursement pathways, evaluation frameworks increasingly highlight the importance of patient-centered outcome measures (PCOMs). The evaluation of digital health applications requires metrics that extend beyond clinical efficacy to include patient-centered outcomes. These outcomes reflect dimensions such as quality of life, functional capacity, and symptom relief that are directly relevant to patients' daily lives. Traditional clinical trials often rely on surrogate endpoints, yet evidence suggests that patient-reported outcome measures (PROMs) and patient-reported experience measures (PREMs) provide a more comprehensive assessment of digital interventions [23].

International frameworks, such as the Patient-Reported Outcomes Measurement Information System (PROMIS) and the EQ-5D instrument, have demonstrated feasibility in capturing subjective health states across different conditions [24, 25]. Integrating such tools into the assessment of DiGA ensures that reimbursement decisions reflect not only cost and safety but also the tangible benefits perceived by patients. This approach aligns with international trends in value-based healthcare, where outcomes that matter to patients are considered the benchmark for innovation [26].

From a methodological perspective, embedding PCOMs into DiGA evaluations presents both opportunities and challenges. On the one hand, digital tools can streamline data collection through in-app questionnaires and passive monitoring, enabling real-time outcome assessment. On the other hand, variation in digital literacy, response biases, and data security concerns require careful consideration to maintain validity and trust. Nevertheless, applying PCOMs strengthens the link between innovation and patient well-being, ensuring that DiGA are not evaluated solely as technological products but as integral components of patient-centered care pathways.

The evolution of DiGA demonstrates how digital health applications can move from isolated pilot projects to system-wide reimbursement and integration. Three key lessons emerge. First, legal entitlement is decisive: without the DVG, pilots would likely have remained fragmented and unequal. Second, infrastructure integration matters: linking DiGA with the eRezept and ePA is essential for sustainability and outcome-based pricing. Third, market sustainability is fragile: while DiGA have enabled innovation, the combination of high evidence requirements and repayment obligations threatens smaller providers. Germany's experience illustrates both the possibilities and pitfalls of institutionalizing digital therapeutics, and its durability will depend on balancing patient-centered access, robust evidence, and payer sustainability.

11.5 Patterns and Challenges in the Utilization of DiGA by Insured Populations

By the end of 2024, nearly one million activation codes for digital health applications (DiGA) had been issued, yet adoption remains highly heterogeneous across demographic groups, therapeutic areas, and access channels [4]. Analyses reveal that women make up the majority of users, with the highest uptake among individuals aged 50 to 64 years. Younger adults between 18 and 34 as well as older adults above 65 show substantially lower participation. These patterns are partly explained by morbidity profiles, since middle-aged adults are more likely to suffer from chronic conditions such as depression, back pain, or metabolic disorders. Younger groups, despite their digital affinity, tend to have less medical need, while older populations face barriers of digital literacy, device access, and usability [6, 7, 21].

The indication-specific distribution of DiGA appears consistent with the demographic profile. Mental health applications dominate overall usage, followed by musculoskeletal and metabolic disorders [4, 27]. The strong uptake in mental health reflects high demand and the suitability of digital cognitive-behavioral interventions for remote delivery. By contrast, adoption in multimorbid or somatic conditions remains limited, highlighting difficulties in integrating DiGA into more complex treatment regimens [21, 27].

Patient access occurs predominantly via prescriptions from physicians and psychotherapists. Surveys indicate that many providers remain cautious, citing concerns about time investment, integration into practice routines, and uncertainty about patient adherence [27]. Direct requests to insurers account for only a small fraction of activations. Intended to facilitate patient autonomy, this route is impeded by procedural bureaucracy (e.g., medical certificates) and by variation in approval practices across insurers, which in turn generates delays in the distribution of activation codes [4].

Experiences reported by patients show both benefits and limitations. Many users value the flexibility and discretion of DiGA, particularly in sensitive areas such as mental health, and report improvements in motivation and self-management [21, 27]. At the same time, elevated dropout rates have been observed. A substantial share of patients discontinue after only a few weeks, citing declining motivation, lack of support, or technical barriers [28, 29]. For long-term conditions such as obesity or diabetes, these adherence problems undermine the potential for lasting health gains. This suggests that DiGA may be most effective when embedded in blended care models rather than as isolated digital interventions [30, 31].

Equity of access remains a pressing challenge. While all insured persons are formally entitled to DiGA, actual use is strongly influenced by education, socioeconomic status, and digital literacy [6, 7]. Patients with lower income or language barriers encounter difficulties in onboarding and navigating app content, creating a second-level digital divide that risks reproducing existing health inequalities [32, 33]. Addressing these disparities will require targeted outreach strategies, user-friendly app design, and multilingual support [34, 35].

Addressing these challenges requires not only broader access but also strategies to sustain patient engagement over time. Sustained engagement with DiGA represents one of the most critical determinants of their long-term effectiveness. Evidence from early pilots shows that many patients discontinue use within the first weeks, limiting potential health benefits despite initial uptake [20, 21]. This pattern mirrors findings in other digital health contexts, where dropout rates of 40–60% after three months are not uncommon [28, 29]. Addressing adherence is therefore essential for ensuring that DiGA deliver measurable improvements in patient outcomes rather than transient effects.

Several strategies have been proposed to enhance longitudinal engagement. Behavioral design elements such as reminders, feedback loops, and gamification can support daily adherence, while personalized goal setting increases perceived relevance [30]. Moreover, integrating DiGA with professional follow-up, through dashboards accessible to physicians or teleconsultation interfaces, links patient activity to clinical care, reinforcing accountability [31]. Studies also suggest that social support features, including peer communities or caregiver involvement, can mitigate attrition and foster long-term usage [31].

From a patient-centric perspective, adherence depends not only on motivational design but also on usability and contextual fit. Complex onboarding procedures, high cognitive demands, or rigid intervention schedules often reduce engagement, especially among older adults or patients with multiple chronic conditions [33, 34]. Conversely, adaptive algorithms that adjust intensity, content, or feedback to individual preferences show promise in maintaining usage over time [32, 36]. Taken together, patient-centric DiGA must be designed not as short-lived interventions but as sustainable components of chronic care pathways, requiring equal attention to clinical validity and user adherence.

From the perspective of payers, these utilization patterns raise concerns about scalability and efficiency. Limited uptake among certain groups reduces the cost-effectiveness of DiGA as a collective benefit, while inconsistent physician engagement and patient adherence complicate outcome measurement, which is central for the upcoming value-based reimbursement components [4]. Administrative delays in code issuance further undermine patient trust in insurers' digital competence [4].

Addressing these disparities requires a stronger emphasis on equity and usability in DiGA design. Simplified interfaces, multilingual support, and targeted outreach can reduce barriers for vulnerable populations, thereby aligning digital health more closely with patient-centric care principles [6, 7, 34]. Special attention is needed for older adults, patients with complex chronic conditions, and individuals with limited digital literacy. Tailored interventions—such as adaptive feedback, integration with caregiver support, and training resources—help ensure that digital applications do not widen existing inequalities but instead contribute to more inclusive and equitable healthcare delivery [33, 35].

Yet, even the most engaging design features cannot compensate for limited digital health literacy, which remains a critical barrier to equitable uptake. Digital health literacy goes beyond the technical ability to operate an app; it includes the capacity to access, understand, and critically evaluate health information in order to make informed decisions. Low digital health literacy has repeatedly been linked to reduced adoption and weaker adherence, particularly among older adults, socioeconomically disadvantaged groups, and patients with multimorbidity [6, 7, 32]. Without targeted interventions, DiGA risk reinforcing existing inequalities rather than mitigating them.

Validated instruments such as the Digital Health Literacy Instrument (DHLI) and the eHealth Literacy Scale (eHEALS) have provided systematic ways to measure these skills [33, 34]. European studies reveal marked disparities: younger, higher-educated users consistently score higher, while older adults and individuals with limited formal education report significantly lower competencies [35]. These findings underline the importance of addressing digital skills as a precondition for effective and patient-centered use of DiGA.

Practical strategies to improve digital health literacy include step-by-step onboarding tutorials, intuitive navigation with low cognitive load, and multilingual support functions. Collaborative models with patient advocacy groups and community health workers have shown potential to increase confidence and sustained use, as they provide personalized guidance and peer-to-peer learning opportunities [36]. Ultimately, enhancing digital health literacy is not a peripheral issue but a central element of patient-centric digital transformation. Only when patients are adequately empowered to navigate and apply digital health information can DiGA realize their full potential in equitable and sustainable care delivery.

In summary, utilization of DiGA in Germany demonstrates their potential to improve access and empower patients, particularly in mental health. At the same time, uneven demographic distribution, barriers in direct insurer access, high dropout rates, and social inequalities indicate that DiGA have not yet achieved their full integrative potential. For sustainable impact, greater attention must be paid to equity, long-term adherence, and supportive structures that connect digital therapeutics with routine care.

11.6 Reimbursement Mechanisms and Payer Perspectives on DiGA Coverage

Reimbursement structures determine whether digital health applications can be sustainably integrated into statutory health systems. The German DiGA model illustrates both innovative mechanisms and structural risks. Central to this framework is a dynamic pricing system in which manufacturers initially set prices freely during the first twelve months after listing. Thereafter, prices are negotiated with the GKV-Spitzenverband, the National Association of Statutory Health Insurance Funds, and applied retrospectively. This mechanism ensures rapid access for patients but introduces financial risks for smaller manufacturers, who may face repayment obligations if negotiated tariffs fall below initial prices. While this secures budgetary control for payers, it has contributed to insolvencies among DiGA providers, reflecting the broader challenge in aligning innovative capacity with fiscal constraints [22, 26].

Physician participation remains a key factor, as the majority of DiGA are accessed through prescriptions rather than direct patient applications. For each prescription, physicians receive a flat-rate remuneration of €7.64, which is included in the national reimbursement catalogue (EBM). This compensation is intended to acknowledge the associated administrative effort [18]. From the perspective of payers, such restrained remuneration supports cost containment and mitigates the risk of overutilization. However, survey data indicate that providers often regard the fee as insufficient, which may contribute to limited diffusion [27].

Beyond financial considerations, physicians remain central to the successful integration of DiGA into routine care. Their involvement is guided primarily by professional responsibility to ensure evidence-based, patient-centered treatment rather than by remuneration alone. When digital applications are presented as tools that support rather than replace clinical judgment, acceptance among both providers and patients is enhanced [7, 8]. Training and institutional support further shape how physicians engage with digital tools. Providers who are equipped to explain benefits and limitations of DiGA can better contextualize their use within individual care plans, strengthening patient trust and adherence. Empirical analyses of patient perspectives suggest that such professional guidance is decisive for sustained utilization [27].

A major strategic innovation is the introduction of outcome-based reimbursement. From 2026 onward, at least 20% of the reimbursement will be linked to real-world effectiveness indicators, measured through Anwendungsbegleitende Erfolgsmessung (AbEM) [5]. Insurers welcome this as a step toward value-based healthcare, but manufacturers express concern about the validity of metrics and the administrative burden of data collection. Patients may ultimately benefit if reimbursement aligns more directly with demonstrated outcomes, but only if evaluation methods capture meaningful health improvements [23, 26].

International comparisons highlight alternative approaches. France employs the PECAN procedure, offering temporary reimbursement for twelve months while requiring evaluation of benefit by the Haute Autorité de Santé [9]. Belgium applies the mHealth Belgium pyramid, a staged certification model linking reimbursement to safety and interoperability compliance [10]. In the United Kingdom, NHS reimbursement is based on procurement processes guided by NICE evidence standards, without separate remuneration for physicians [11]. The United States provides FDA regulatory approval but leaves reimbursement fragmented across Medicare and private insurers, with limited outcome-based contracts piloted [12, 13].

Table 11.2 summarizes these reimbursement mechanisms across Germany, France, Belgium, the United Kingdom, and the United States, comparing evidence requirements, physician remuneration, and outcome-based components. Beyond institutional mechanisms, a patient-centric perspective highlights how different national systems integrate usability, equity, and patient involvement into digital health strategies. In France, the PECAN procedure requires not only demonstration of clinical efficacy but also evidence of real-world usability, thereby emphasizing patient experience alongside safety and effectiveness [9]. Belgium's mHealth pyramid goes one step further by embedding co-creation: patient associations are systematically involved in the evaluation process, ensuring that applications respond to everyday needs rather than only to regulatory criteria [19]. The United Kingdom has developed its NHS framework with a strong focus on transparency for patients, providing easily understandable summaries of app functions, data use, and evidence standards [11]. This emphasis on communication enhances trust and facilitates informed decision-making, particularly for individuals with lower health literacy [6, 7]. In the United States, by contrast, reimbursement pilots under Medicare and private insurers have been more fragmented, often limiting patient access to specific populations or conditions [13]. Although pilot projects have highlighted potential benefits, the absence of standardized patient-centered outcome reporting constrains scalability.

Table 11.2 Reimbursement mechanisms across different countries

Country	Evidence requirements	Physician remuneration	Outcome-based components
Germany	RCTs or comparative studies required within 12 months of provisional listing	Flat-rate fee (€7.64) via EBM code	≥20% outcome-linked from 2026 (AbEM)
France	Clinical or organizational benefit required (HAS evaluation)	No specific remuneration; integrated into physician fee schedules	Planned incorporation of real-world evidence in revisions
Belgium	Certification at staged levels, no fixed RCT requirement	No dedicated physician fee; system-level reimbursement	Outcome-based mechanisms not yet defined
UK (NHS)	Evidence required via NICE standards framework	No extra remuneration; included in NHS contracts	Focus on safety and clinical validation, not outcome-based pricing
USA	FDA approval for safety/efficacy, no reimbursement guarantee	Varies by insurer; no standard remuneration	Outcome-based contracts piloted by private insurers

Taken together, these comparisons suggest that international approaches differ not only in reimbursement structures but also in the degree to which patient perspectives are embedded in evaluation and communication. While Germany has pioneered entitlement-based access through the DiGA pathway, other countries highlight complementary dimensions: usability (France), co-creation (Belgium), transparency (UK), and accessibility (USA). Incorporating these elements may help refine Germany's model toward a more comprehensive patient-centered strategy, ensuring that regulatory innovation translates into tangible improvements for diverse patient populations.

As Table 11.2 shows, Germany is distinctive in combining early market access with retrospective tariff corrections and a planned outcome-based component. France emphasizes stringent evidence requirements, Belgium prioritizes layered certification, the NHS focuses on centralized procurement and safety standards, and the United States illustrates the challenges of fragmented reimbursement. Each model reflects different trade-offs between payer security, provider incentives, and manufacturer sustainability. For Germany, the long-term sustainability of DiGA reimbursement will depend on balancing payer safeguards with stronger provider engagement and more predictable conditions for manufacturers.

Looking ahead, patient-centric care can be further strengthened by value-based reimbursement models. Rather than linking payment to utilization volumes, such approaches tie coverage to improvements in patient-relevant outcomes, including quality of life, symptom relief, and functional capacity [23, 25, 26]. This alignment encourages manufacturers to design digital applications that generate sustainable benefits for patients. For payers, outcome-based contracts also mitigate the risk of financing tools with limited clinical impact. By focusing on evidence of effectiveness and patient engagement, reimbursement mechanisms can promote innovations that demonstrably improve care delivery. In this way, value-based care links economic considerations to the principle of patient-centeredness, ensuring that financial structures directly serve the well-being of patients [23, 26].

11.7 Conclusion

The German DiGA framework demonstrates how digital health applications can be incorporated into statutory care, but it also reveals persistent structural challenges such as uneven utilization, high dropout rates, and financial risks for smaller providers. Ensuring transparency, meaningful consent, and safeguards against bias is essential for patient trust and long-term acceptance of digital health applications.

Utilization remains concentrated among women in midlife, while younger, older, and socioeconomically disadvantaged groups are underrepresented. Equity must be addressed so that digital transformation reduces, rather than reinforces, existing divides in age, gender, and socioeconomic status.

Physician involvement continues to be a cornerstone of DiGA implementation. While remuneration acknowledges administrative effort, physicians' participation is decisive, guided by their professional work and their ability to contextualize digital tools within evidence-based patient care.

International comparisons illustrate that reimbursement mechanisms vary across Europe and beyond, but Germany remains the first country to combine regulatory approval with systematic reimbursement. Partnerships between industry, payers, and patient groups can enhance usability and ensure that digital tools reflect real patient needs.

Current reimbursement safeguards budgetary control but also create tensions between innovation and financial sustainability. Future reimbursement strategies should increasingly link coverage to patient-relevant outcomes, aligning financial mechanisms with the principle of patient-centered care.

For the further development of DiGA, three factors are decisive: first, building patient trust through transparency and equitable access; second, ensuring physician involvement based on professional ethos and evidence-based guidance; and third, implementing value-based reimbursement models that reward measurable improvements in patient outcomes. Together, these elements form the foundation for sustainable, patient-centered digital health integration.

References

1. World Health Organization. Global strategy on digital health 2020–2025. Geneva: WHO; 2021.
2. Bundesinstitut für Arzneimittel und Medizinprodukte (BfArM). DiGA-Verzeichnis. Bonn: BfArM; 2024.
3. Bundesministerium für Gesundheit. Digitale-Versorgung-Gesetz (DVG). Berlin: BMG; 2019.
4. Spitzenverband Digitale Gesundheitsversorgung (SVDGV). DiGA-Report 2024. Berlin: SVDGV; 2024.
5. Bundesministerium für Gesundheit. Digital-Gesetz (DigiG). Berlin: BMG; 2024.
6. Kruse CS, Stein A, Thomas H, Kaur H. The digital divide in healthcare: barriers and opportunities. J Med Internet Res. 2018;20(1):e17.
7. Barello S, Triberti S, Graffigna G. Digital health literacy and patient engagement: implications for adoption of digital therapeutics. Front Public Health. 2021;9:690975.
8. Bundesärztekammer (BÄK). Ärztliche Haltung zu Digitalen Gesundheitsanwendungen. Berlin: BÄK; 2022.
9. Haute Autorité de Santé (HAS). PECAN procedure for digital medical devices. Paris: HAS; 2023.
10. mHealth Belgium. Validation pyramid for mobile health apps. Brussels: Belgian Federal Public Service; 2019–2022.
11. National Institute for Health and Care Excellence (NICE). Evidence standards framework for digital health technologies. London: NICE; 2019–2024.
12. U.S. Food and Drug Administration (FDA). Digital Health Center of Excellence. Silver Spring: FDA; 2024.
13. Centers for Medicare & Medicaid Services (CMS). Remote Patient Monitoring reimbursement guidance. Baltimore: CMS; 2024.
14. European Commission. European Health Data Space (EHDS). Brussels: EC; 2022.
15. European Union. Artificial Intelligence Act. Brussels: Publications Office of the EU; 2024.
16. Bundesministerium für Gesundheit. Digitalisierungsstrategie für das Gesundheitswesen und die Pflege. Berlin: BMG; 2023.
17. DAK-Gesundheit. Pilotprojekt App-basierte DiGA-Verordnung. Hamburg: DAK; 2023.
18. Kassenärztliche Bundesvereinigung (KBV). Einheitlicher Bewertungsmaßstab (EBM) und Integration digitaler Gesundheitsanwendungen. Berlin: KBV; 2023.

19. OECD. Partnerships for digital health innovation: co-creation and validation frameworks. Paris: OECD; 2022.
20. Albrecht UV, et al. Digital health pilots in Germany: lessons from pre-DVG initiatives. J Med Internet Res. 2019;21(9):e14990.
21. Gerke S, Stern AD, Minssen T. Germany's digital health reforms in the COVID-19 era: lessons and opportunities for other countries. NPJ Digit Med. 2020;3:94.
22. Die WELT. Warum Start-ups mit Apps auf Rezept so häufig scheitern. Berlin: Axel Springer; 2023.
23. Black N. Patient reported outcome measures could help transform healthcare. BMJ. 2013;346:f167.
24. Cella D, et al. The patient-reported outcomes measurement information system (PROMIS). Med Care. 2007;45(5 Suppl 1):S3–11.
25. EuroQol Group. EuroQol—a new facility for the measurement of health-related quality of life. Health Policy. 1990;16(3):199–208.
26. Porter ME. What is value in health care? N Engl J Med. 2010;363(26):2477–81.
27. Swoboda W, et al. Utilization of digital health applications in German statutory health insurance: an empirical analysis. Health Policy. 2023;127(5):560–8.
28. Eysenbach G. The law of attrition. J Med Internet Res. 2005;7(1):e11.
29. Yardley L, et al. Understanding and promoting effective engagement with digital behavior change interventions. Am J Prev Med. 2016;51(5):833–42.
30. Kelders SM, et al. Persuasive system design does matter: a systematic review of adherence to web-based interventions. J Med Internet Res. 2012;14(6):e152.
31. Mohr DC, et al. Barriers and facilitators to engagement with digital mental health interventions. BMC Psychiatry. 2017;17:258.
32. Nahum-Shani I, et al. Just-in-time adaptive interventions (JITAI): an organizing framework. Ann Behav Med. 2018;52(6):446–62.
33. van der Vaart R, et al. Development and validation of the Digital Health Literacy Instrument (DHLI). J Med Internet Res. 2017;19(1):e27.
34. Norman CD, Skinner HA. eHEALS: the eHealth literacy scale. J Med Internet Res. 2006;8(4):e27.
35. Hargittai E, et al. Digital inequality and older adults: internet skills, health information seeking, and health literacy. J Gerontol B Psychol Sci Soc Sci. 2019;74(5):821–31.
36. Struik LL, et al. Digital health literacy interventions for vulnerable populations: a scoping review. J Public Health. 2021;43(1):e90–e102.

Part VI

Transforming Care Models: Digital Innovation in Residential and Home Settings

12 Digital Transformation in Long-Term: Perspectives from Nursing Practice

Vera Antonia Büchner

Demographic change is leading to a steadily aging society. By the end of 2023, 5.7 million people in Germany were in need of long-term care under the Social Code Book XI [1]. Projections estimate an increase to between 6.8 and 7.6 million by 2055. The shortage of skilled nursing staff is already one of the greatest challenges facing the German health care system. According to the Pflege-Report 2019 [2], depending on the scenario, between 130,000 and more than 300,000 additional professional nurses will be required by 2035. These shortages result primarily from demographic change, rising care needs, and age-related retirements, while the number of newly trained nurses will not cover demand. Moreover, the high workload contributes to dropouts during training and to nurses leaving the profession, thereby exacerbating the shortage.

Against this background, digitalization is often discussed as a central response to existing care gaps. Digital technologies can reduce the burden on nursing practice, make workflows more efficient, and improve quality of care. However, in order to fully realize this potential, their introduction and use must be carefully managed. In addition to technical infrastructure and clear strategies, three central prerequisites are required: organizational digital readiness, meaning the capacity to integrate innovations into existing structures; digital maturity, reflecting the stage of development and strategic anchoring of digital transformation within the organization; and digital competencies among staff and leadership, enabling the reflective, safe, and effective use of technologies.

This chapter focuses on the digital transformation of long-term residential care facilities. Following a categorization of digital innovations in nursing and a discussion of the foundations for successful implementation, Section 12.1 analyzes the opportunities and challenges of digital innovations in long-term care. Section 12.2 examines the transferability of concepts of digital readiness and maturity to the care

V. A. Büchner (✉)
Nuremberg Institute of Technology Georg Simon Ohm, Nürnberg, Germany
e-mail: veraantonia.buechner@th-nuernberg.de

S. Scholz et al. (eds.), *Advancements in Digital Health and Care*,
https://doi.org/10.1007/978-3-032-16837-5_12

sector, with particular emphasis on organizational prerequisites, strategic governance, and leadership behavior. Finally, Sect. 12.3 highlights the digital competencies of staff and leadership, which are considered key qualifications for successful digital transformation. This underlines that digital competencies are an essential component of professional nursing and must be developed systematically at the individual, organizational, and leadership levels.

12.1 Digital Innovations in Long-Term Residential Care: Opportunities and Constraints

Digital innovations are becoming increasingly important in long-term residential care. They encompass a wide range of applications, from digital documentation and communication platforms to sensor-based monitoring systems and robotic assistance solutions. The common goal of these technologies is to relieve nursing staff, improve quality and safety of care, and promote the independence and participation of residents in long-term care facilities. In doing so, digital solutions address central challenges of long-term care such as staff shortages, rising care needs, and the demand for high-quality services. At the same time, however, the implementation of such technologies faces numerous barriers. Issues of financing, data protection, and interoperability, as well as acceptance problems among staff, residents, and family members, pose significant challenges.

12.1.1 Foundations of Successful Implementation in Long-Term Care

In care-related areas, digital solutions primarily include systems for nursing documentation and information management. Electronic documentation systems are increasingly replacing paper-based procedures, enabling faster, more structured, and often legally reliable recording of care processes. In addition, monitoring systems such as wearables continuously measure vital signs, detect abnormalities, and automatically transmit them. These technologies facilitate the monitoring of residents, reduce sources of error, and allow for quicker responses to critical situations in long-term care facilities [3].

In non-care areas, robotic systems are being tested primarily for household and logistical tasks. Robots can transport laundry or distribute materials more efficiently. This automation relieves nursing staff of physically demanding routine tasks, enabling them to focus more on their core nursing responsibilities. At the same time, systems for social interaction are being introduced, such as social robots or digital communication platforms. They aim to reduce loneliness, involve relatives, and provide residents with new opportunities for leisure activities [4].

Regardless of the specific technology used, the successful implementation of such systems requires careful preparation with respect to ethical, legal [especially data protection under the General Data Protection Regulation (GDPR)], social, nursing practice, economic, and technical issues and prerequisites [5].

A number of technical requirements must be met: a powerful IT infrastructure with stable network coverage, appropriate end devices, and secure server solutions are indispensable. Insufficient Wi-Fi coverage or inadequate equipment quickly results in systems not being used or in acceptance problems. Equally important is interoperability: only if systems can communicate with one another can media discontinuities be avoided and data used efficiently. Missing interfaces to the telematics infrastructure or incompatible software solutions are currently among the greatest obstacles to digitalization in long-term care facilities [6].

In addition to technical foundations, legal and ethical issues play a decisive role. Long-term care facilities work with highly sensitive health data, the protection of which under the GDPR has the highest priority. Therefore, data protection and IT security concepts must already be developed during the preparation phase. Liability issues also need to be clarified. Financing is equally crucial, as digital systems involve high acquisition and maintenance costs. Another prerequisite for success is the involvement of staff. Studies show that the acceptance of digital technologies depends heavily on the early participation of nursing professionals [2, 3, 6].

In addition to these practical foundations, it can be useful to apply structured frameworks to analyze barriers to implementation. One example is the Nonadoption, Abandonment, Scale-up, Spread, and Sustainability (NASSS) framework [7], which considers factors such as NASSS of digital technologies. It highlights why digital solutions may fail in practice despite technical feasibility or strategic planning. A more detailed discussion is provided in Sect. 12.2.2.

12.1.2 Opportunities of Digital Innovations in Long-Term Care

The digital transformation offers long-term care facilities a wide range of opportunities that affect both work processes and the quality of care. A central potential lies in relieving the nursing staff. Electronic documentation systems enable standardized and faster recording of information. Automated collection of vital signs reduces the time required for routine checks. Digital scheduling or route planning software optimizes staff deployment and workflows. Robotic systems that handle internal transport reduce the physical strain on caregivers. This relief allows nurses to dedicate more time to their core nursing tasks and direct care. The aim of these developments is to support nursing practice, not to fully substitute it. Frey and Osborne show in their analysis of the automation potential of more than 700 occupational groups that activities with a high proportion of routine tasks are particularly at risk. For elderly care, however, the substitutability potential is low, since complex social interactions, empathy, and situational judgment are central. These skills can hardly be replaced by digital systems so far and underline that digitalization in nursing should be understood not as a replacement but as a support and complement to human work [8].

In addition, digital technologies can improve the quality of care and patient safety. Monitoring systems that continuously record vital signs help detect deterioration in health conditions at an early stage. Smart mattresses or sensors can prevent falls or report them in time. Digital medication systems minimize the risk of prescription and administration errors by cross-checking medication plans and automatically alerting nursing staff.

Another advantage lies in the improvement of communication and transparency. Digital platforms allow relatives to gain insight into the care situation of their family members at any time. Video calls create opportunities to involve relatives more closely, even when they live far away. Within the facility, digital handover tools facilitate the exchange of information between shifts and professional groups. This reduces misunderstandings and, in turn, increases the quality of care.

Digital innovations also contribute to the quality of life and participation of residents. Social robots or interactive assistance systems can expand leisure activities, support activation measures, or initiate conversations. Ambient assisted living technologies strengthen independence, for example, by reminding residents to take their medication. These applications can not only improve care but also reduce loneliness and promote social participation.

Moreover, digitalization can enhance the attractiveness of the nursing profession. A work environment that meaningfully integrates digital systems is perceived as modern and future-oriented. Nurses who are relieved by digital support report higher job satisfaction. For a sector heavily affected by staff shortages, this can be a decisive advantage [2].

12.1.3 Constraints of Digital Innovations in Long-Term Care

As great as the potential of digital innovations in elderly care may be, the challenges and limitations that can restrict the success of digital technologies in long-term residential care are equally numerous.

One of the central barriers is financing. Digital systems are associated with high acquisition and ongoing costs. While research and funding projects can facilitate initial adoption as short-term support, sustainable refinancing models are often lacking. Facilities are therefore faced with the challenge of developing long-term investment strategies that take ongoing costs into account. For many institutions, this represents a significant hurdle, as they are already operating under considerable financial pressure [5].

Another problem concerns the acceptance of technologies. Nursing staff sometimes respond with skepticism when they fear that technology will complicate their work or eventually replace them. Residents and relatives also express reservations, particularly regarding data protection. Different levels of competence can lead to risk of digital exclusion, especially when older employees or residents have difficulties handling digital tools. Studies show that technological stress (“technostress”) arises less from the technologies themselves than from problematic implementation, for example, due to insufficient training or lack of participation [9].

Nursing professionals must have the opportunity to contribute their perspectives in the context of co-creation, so that technologies can be adapted to their working reality. Equally decisive is continuous training and competence development that enables staff to use the systems safely and reflectively. Without such support, uncertainty and overload arise (see Sect. 12.3).

Another major issue is the lack of interoperability. Many facilities use isolated software solutions that cannot communicate with each other. This leads to media discontinuities and redundant documentation. Connection to the telematics infrastructure is still not comprehensively ensured. Standardized interfaces are missing, which makes the integration of new systems more difficult.

Data protection and data security are also critical issues. Working with highly sensitive health data requires the highest security standards. Uncertainty about responsibilities or access rights often leads to skepticism among residents and relatives. Questions of data sovereignty, i.e., who decides on the use and disclosure of data remain largely unresolved.

Structural conditions are also problematic. The shortage of skilled staff persists and is exacerbated by additional demands for digital competencies. Facilities must not only recruit and retain staff but also provide continuous training. In addition, the implementation of the Nursing Professions Act requires considerable resources and binds attention that would otherwise be needed for digitalization.

Finally, ethical tensions must not be overlooked. An overly technology-oriented approach carries the risk of dehumanization. Nursing is more than process optimization; it is characterized by empathy, relationships, and situational judgment. Here, tensions arise between efficiency and personal care, which must always be considered when implementing new technologies [3].

Table 12.1 summarizes the key opportunities and constraints of digital innovations in long-term residential care and provides a basis for the subsequent discussion.

Overall, it becomes clear that the digital transformation in nursing offers considerable opportunities, but these can only be realized if the necessary foundations for implementation are in place and the existing barriers are consistently addressed. Digital innovations in long-term residential care can relieve staff, improve care quality, enhance residents' quality of life, and increase the attractiveness of the profession. At the same time, however, significant barriers remain in terms of financing, interoperability, data protection, acceptance, and ethical implications. The opportunities and risks presented demonstrate that digital transformation does not occur solely at the technical level but constitutes a comprehensive socio-technical and cultural change process at both the organizational and employee levels in long-term care facilities. This makes it clear that digitalization should not be understood as a one-time project but as a continuous process that can only succeed under appropriate infrastructural conditions [10].

This change affects structures, strategies, processes, and organizational culture within facilities and must therefore be regarded as a profound organizational development process [11]. This becomes particularly evident in communication, which in many facilities is hampered by parallel paper-based and digital documentation, impeding the flow of information. At the same time, it is clear that digitalization is

Table 12.1 Opportunities and constraints of digital innovations in long-term residential care

Opportunities	Constraints
Relief of nursing staff through digital documentation, automated vital sign recording, robotic logistics systems	High investment and operating costs, lack of sustainable refinancing models
Improvement of care quality (e.g., through monitoring, fall sensors, medication management)	Lack of interoperability between systems, heterogeneous IT landscapes, insufficient connection to telematics infrastructure
Enhanced communication and transparency (digital handovers, family portals, video calls)	Data protection and security risks, unresolved questions of data sovereignty
Increased quality of life and participation through social robots, assistance systems, and activation offers	Low acceptance among staff, residents, and relatives; risk of technostress
Data-based care and service planning through systematic evaluation of care data	Staff shortage, additional need for training and qualifications
Increased attractiveness of the nursing profession through modern work environments and relief from routine tasks	Ethical tensions, risk of dehumanization due to excessive technology orientation

Own presentation based on [2, 3, 6, 9, 10]

redefining leadership qualities: leadership, management, and communication are taking place under the conditions of digital transformation and must actively shape change. Staff are also challenged, as the acquisition of digital competencies—such as handling AI-based systems—is a prerequisite for acceptance and successful use. It is crucial that both organizations and employees are enabled to participate in the transformation process through continuous support from leadership, transparent communication, and participatory involvement.

Thus, digital transformation must be understood as a change process that requires a reassessment of resources, skills, and processes at the organizational level, while also transforming attitudes, competencies, and role models at the individual level. This dual perspective is further elaborated in the following sections on organizational digital maturity (Sect. 12.2) and digital competencies of staff and leadership (Sect. 12.3).

12.2 Assessing Organizational Digital Readiness and Maturity in Long-Term Care

The successful implementation of digital transformation in long-term residential care largely depends on the organizational conditions of the institutions. In addition to technical infrastructure and financial resources, increasing attention is being paid to digital readiness and digital maturity. These concepts make it possible to systematically assess the extent to which organizations are capable of implementing digital technologies and embedding them sustainably into structures, processes, and culture. The following sections define the key terms (Sect. 12.2.1), present existing models for measurement (Sect. 12.2.2), and discuss their transferability to the context of long-term care (Sect. 12.2.3).

12.2.1 Digital Readiness and Digital Maturity: Concepts and Distinctions

The terms digital readiness and digital maturity have become established in organizational research and today represent central analytical categories for assessing the digital development status of companies, facilities, or institutions. Both concepts are closely related but address different perspectives in the digital transformation process.

Digital readiness describes the degree of attitude, capability, and organizational preparedness of an institution with regard to the introduction and use of digital technologies. It encompasses technical and infrastructural prerequisites, strategic capacity to act, and individual and collective competencies required to integrate digital innovations into work and care processes. Typically, it is an ex ante perspective: the key question is whether an organization is "ready to begin digitalization." This includes the availability of stable IT infrastructures, the provision of financial and human resources, and an organizational culture that allows for change. An example from nursing would be a home care service assessing whether its employees are sufficiently trained to use a new documentation system.

Digital maturity, on the other hand, refers to the achieved level of development of an organization within the process of digital transformation, that is, the degree and depth of integration of digital processes, technologies, and structures. The term is understood as a state in which digital technologies are not only introduced but firmly embedded in core processes (strategies, structures, and organizational cultures) and accompanied by profound structural and cultural changes [12, 13]. Operationalization typically takes place through maturity models that assess the level of development across several dimensions—such as technology, processes, culture, competencies, and strategy [14]. This perspective is ex post or concurrent: for example, a nursing home might reach an intermediate level of maturity if digital documentation is already established but teleconsultations or AI-supported assistance systems are still lacking.

In summary, digital readiness evaluates the ability and preparedness for digital change, while digital maturity captures the achieved level of integration and transformation. Both concepts are complementary and allow for a differentiated analysis of organizational digitalization processes in long-term care.

Applied to health care, it is assumed that higher maturity levels are associated with more efficient processes and improved care outcomes. This applies both to the quality of nursing services and to organizational performance, for example, through streamlined workflows, fewer media discontinuities, and better use of data [15–17]. Readiness and maturity models are therefore essential instruments for systematically assessing the state of digital transformation, guiding investments, and securing competitiveness and sustainability in the long term [18].

Building on these conceptual distinctions, the next section (Sect. 12.2.2) introduces existing models for assessing digital maturity. These models provide structured approaches to evaluating the degree of digital development across multiple dimensions. They differ in scope, methodology, and applicability, and their benefits and limitations must be carefully considered, particularly when transferring them to the specific context of long-term care.

12.2.2 Models for Measuring Digital Maturity

In recent years, numerous models have been developed to measure the digital maturity of organizations and enterprises. Their purpose is to support institutions in determining their stage of digital development. However, the scientific evidence on the quality and effectiveness of existing models remains limited. Many approaches are associated with high time and resource requirements, methodological uncertainty regarding reliability and validity, or biases caused by self-assessment [15, 17]. In addition, capturing the complexity of digital transformation in standardized instruments without overburdening organizations remains a major challenge. Cresswell et al. emphasize the high costs of data collection, questions of measurement accuracy, and issues of long-term comparability [17].

Flott et al., in a systematic review, identified five core dimensions of digital maturity: evaluation methodology, resources and capabilities, use, interoperability, and outcomes. Methodological approaches and usage aspects have been studied most frequently, whereas outcome dimensions have so far been underrepresented [18].

Duncan et al. expand this perspective by highlighting dimensions such as education and training, knowledge management, individual competencies, and technology use. This illustrates that digital maturity encompasses not only technology and processes but is closely linked to organizational learning. Moreover, they argue that digital maturity should ultimately be measured against the goals of the Quadruple Aim: improved patient outcomes, promotion of population health, cost reduction, and higher professional satisfaction [19].

Particularly widespread are the models of the Healthcare Information and Management Systems Society (HIMSS), most notably the Electronic Medical Record Adoption Model (EMRAM), which classifies hospitals in seven stages according to their adoption of electronic medical records [20]. Other models include O-EMRAM (outpatient), CCMM (continuity of care), and DIAM (digital imaging). These are considered international standards, but they have been criticized for being too technology-centric while neglecting organizational and cultural factors [12].

The WHO and OECD have also published frameworks that emphasize interoperability, data analytics, and competencies. These models underline the importance of structured assessments for steering digital transformation projects but at the same time demonstrate that technological evaluations must always be complemented by organizational and human dimensions [16, 21].

In Germany, the DigitalRadar was introduced under the Krankenhauszukunftsgesetz (KHZG) as a comprehensive instrument. It is based on 234 items, covers seven dimensions (including IT infrastructure, clinical processes, data management, patient engagement, and telemedicine). The results revealed significant deficits in interoperability and process integration, while baseline technologies were more strongly developed [22].

In addition, a maturity model was developed for German public health authorities, comprising eight dimensions (e.g., infrastructure, data protection, strategic management, staff qualification), enabling targeted planning of digital strategies [23].

12.2.3 Transferability of Existing Models to Long-Term Care

So far, no validated maturity models exist for long-term care. Most existing approaches originate from the hospital context and can only be transferred to a limited extent, as structures, resources, and processes differ significantly in key respects [17]. Long-term care facilities operate with smaller teams, have limited financial resources, and rely heavily on relatives and informal caregivers; these aspects are hardly taken into account by existing models.

Against this background, Savic and Büchner aim for the first time to systematically focus on digital maturity models for long-term care and to develop a digital maturity care model: PflegeDigitalRadar tailored to the requirements of residential and home-based care. The basis is a systematic literature review (856 publications identified). The analysis shows that, in addition to strategy, processes, and interoperability, technological infrastructure can be used as an established dimension. At the same time, greater emphasis must be placed on the digital competencies of professionals and managers [19, 24]. These dimensions will be operationalized in the further research process to enable organizations to make a realistic self-assessment.

Overall, it becomes clear that specific maturity models must be developed for long-term care that equally capture technological, organizational, and personnel aspects. Only in this way can the potentials of digitalization, such as efficiency gains, quality improvements, and sustainable care provision be realized.

The previous discussion also makes it clear that digital maturity cannot be considered in isolation. It is closely linked to the competencies of staff and leadership and requires a parallel cultural transformation. Thus, Sect. 12.3 forms the logical next step: the targeted development of digital competencies in long-term care.

12.3 Developing Digital Competencies in Long-Term Care Staff and Leadership

Digital transformation is fundamentally reshaping nursing practice. In particular, artificial intelligence, robotics, sensor-based assistance systems, and digital documentation and communication solutions open up new possibilities for organizing workflows more efficiently and improving the quality of care for residents in long-term care facilities. At the same time, however, the introduction and use of these technologies confront nursing professionals, organizations, and leadership with profound challenges. Integrating new systems into everyday practice requires not only technical infrastructure and financial resources, but above all competencies that ensure the safe, reflective, and responsible use of digital technologies. Central to this is the systematic development of digital competencies among nursing professionals. Yet digital competencies concern not only individual staff members but also entire institutions and their leadership levels. They therefore represent a systemic construct that can only unfold its impact if developed strategically and in a structured manner across all levels.

12.3.1 Empirical Evidence and Research Findings

In the scientific literature, digital competencies are not reduced to mere technical proficiency but encompass a wide range of skills. These include media literacy, data and information literacy, problem-solving ability, ethical judgment, as well as collaborative and communication skills [25, 26]. The concept of competence serves as a binding frame of reference both in the German education system and in health care. Competence describes the ability to apply knowledge and skills in specific situations, to reflect on actions, and to act autonomously. As early as 2017, the Nursing 4.0 Guidelines emphasized that nursing professionals should acquire basic IT education and specific media literacy during their training. However, given the high dynamics of technical and digital innovation, it is not possible to comprehensively convey all relevant knowledge during initial training. Continuous, modular continuing education concepts are therefore required, targeting different groups and making use of modern teaching and learning methods [27].

For nursing, this means that professionals must be enabled not only to use digital applications, but also to critically assess them, integrate them into their work processes, and evaluate their impact on care, organization, and patient well-being. Digital competencies are thus not merely technical skills but also a matter of communication and ethical reflection.

Research on the acquisition and transfer of digital competencies in nursing has increased significantly in recent years, but remains largely fragmented. Krick et al., for example, show in their review that numerous pilot projects promise positive effects, but evidence of their effectiveness is rarely empirically verifiable. There is therefore still a lack of robust evaluations of the actual benefits of digital care technologies [6]. Seyda et al. examine digital competencies in elderly care compared with the overall economy in Germany. They show that in addition to technical skills, digital communication competencies and an awareness of data protection are also necessary. Barriers are primarily technical problems, lack of training, and insufficient acceptance [28]. In Wales, Havard et al. surveyed nurses about "digital nursing." The results show that nursing professionals have very different ideas of what digital nursing means. Central issues include access, impact on care, specific technologies, and the digital future [29].

The selection of current studies underlines that digital competencies include both technical knowledge and communicative and ethical skills. At the same time, they show that acceptance and successful use can only be achieved through participatory development processes and targeted continuing education.

12.3.2 Dimensions of Digital Competencies

A systematic overview makes it possible to structure digital competencies along three levels: the individual level (employees/nursing professionals), the organizational level (organizations and institutions), and the leadership level [3, 30]. This overview provides a sound basis for designing competence development not as a one-off intervention but in a strategic and systemic manner:

- *Digital understanding and knowledge*
  - *Employees*: technical knowledge, user competence, media and data literacy, problem-solving ability, handling of digital interfaces, willingness to learn
  - *Organizations*: integration of digital technologies into work processes, ensuring IT infrastructure
  - *Leadership*: promotion of digital processes, active use of AI-supported decision-making
- *Digital ethics*
  - *Employees*: data protection awareness, ethical judgment, critical reflection.
  - *Organizations*: establishment of data protection and IT security policies, implementation of ethical standards
  - *Leadership*: role model function, ethical decision-making, communication of values, ensuring fairness and transparency
- *Leading with technology/collaboration*
  - *Employees*: introduction of digital tools into daily work, self-organization, digital communication, teamwork
  - *Organizations*: digital training programs, promotion of teamwork and networking, design of transparent processes
  - *Leadership*: collaboration and co-creation, new leadership models, mentoring and coaching
- *Agility & innovation*
  - *Employees*: adaptability, flexibility, continuous willingness to learn, use of agile methods

  - *Organizations*: capacity for innovation, promotion of agile structures, "new work" approaches, development of an innovation culture
  - *Leadership*: accompanying cultural change, active change management, dealing with resistance and fears
- *Digital attitude and behavior*
  - *Employees*: acceptance, critical thinking, openness, active use of digital solutions
  - *Organizations*: provision and maintenance of user-friendly systems, promotion of the application of digital solutions, creation of suitable framework conditions, support for digital practices
  - *Leadership*: process support, motivation, reduction of fears, support for technology acceptance, communication, role model function
- *Consultation and communication*
  - *Employees*: advising patients and relatives on digital support options
  - *Organizations*: provision of suitable information channels
  - *Leadership*: positioning as a competent partner in the digital care network (see, e.g., [3, 30–35])

This overview highlights that digital competencies cannot be understood in isolation as pertaining to individual nursing professionals but must be embedded in organizational structures and leadership practices.

12.3.3 Success Factors for Digital Transformation and Competence Development

A successful digital transformation is closely linked to organizational development. Wolf-Ostermann & Rothgang show that although digital technologies in nursing hold great potential for reducing workloads and improving quality, their integration often fails due to barriers such as lack of practical applicability, unclear financing, and insufficient evaluation. They emphasize the importance of participatory development, organizational embedding, and sustainable financing [3].

The German Federal Ministry of Labour and Social Affairs (BMAS) and studies by Kubek et al. also highlight that digitalization is not merely a technical project but a comprehensive transformation process that affects work organization, qualification, and leadership equally. Organizational development includes adapting processes, promoting an innovation-friendly culture, and creating a learning-oriented environment. It is therefore not only a framework condition but an active component of digital competence development [34, 35].

The following central success factors can be identified:

- *Leadership competence and change management*: Leaders must formulate a clear digital strategy, communicate it, and accompany its implementation.
- *Participation of nursing practice*: Nursing staff should be involved from the outset in selection and implementation processes to ensure acceptance and relevance.

- *Organizational development*: Digital transformation requires structural adjustments, such as agile work practices and innovation cultures.
- *Learning and error culture:* Mistakes must be understood as learning opportunities. Only then can an open attitude toward new technologies emerge.
- *Communication and transparency:* Clear and continuous communication about opportunities and challenges strengthens trust in digital solutions.

These factors make it clear that digital competencies can only be developed sustainably if they are embedded in a comprehensive, strategically managed organizational development process.

The future of digital competence development in nursing is characterized by several open research questions. Westerman et al. already emphasized that establishing a culture of digital readiness is a key prerequisite [12]. Deficits in digital competencies at all levels not only hinder the introduction of new technologies but also their sustainable integration into digital transformation processes. Santarsiero et al. and Tenggono et al. point to a significant evidence gap: it remains unclear how management qualifications foster the development of dynamic leadership competencies and to what extent these competencies are decisive for the digital readiness of organizations. They stress the need to systematically link management development with competence promotion [36, 37].

Against this background, it becomes evident that digital competencies in nursing are no longer an optional addition but an indispensable part of professional practice. Cheeseman points out that nursing professionals already rely on digital skills in key areas such as digital documentation. Furthermore, the concept of competence must be understood more broadly: digital competence includes technical knowledge, an understanding of data protection, ethical judgment, as well as communicative and collaborative skills [38].

Overall, it becomes clear that digital competencies represent a strategic resource for the future of nursing. At the individual level, they concern technical knowledge, data protection, and ethical judgment; at the organizational level, they relate to integration, infrastructure, and standards; at the leadership level, strategic change management and a culture of digital readiness are decisive. Their development must therefore not take place sporadically but must be systematic, continuous, and sustainable in order to shape the digital transformation of nursing successfully and responsibly.

Digital transformation in nursing is not merely a process of introducing technology, but a complex socio-technical change in which technological innovations, organizational development processes, and cultural shifts are closely intertwined. Its success depends fundamentally on three factors: reliable infrastructure, clear strategic governance, and the targeted involvement and qualification of staff.

Digital technologies such as robotics, AI, or sensor-based assistance systems offer significant potential, for example, to relieve nursing staff, ensure quality of care, and strengthen transparency and participation. At the same time, risks such as digital divide, overload, or ethical tensions must be addressed. What is crucial is an innovation-oriented organizational culture that fosters openness, participation, and a constructive error culture. Leaders play a key role by building trust, promoting acceptance, and actively shaping change processes.

In addition, the digital maturity of institutions is a decisive indicator for successful implementation: it reflects the extent to which technological innovations are integrated into structures, processes, and culture, and whether organizations possess the necessary strategic management capacity.

Sustainable digital transformation also requires digital competencies at all levels: nursing staff need practical application and reflection skills, middle management requires process and coordination competencies, and leadership must provide strategic change management. Strategic change management and a culture of digital readiness are decisive. These competencies must be continuously developed and promoted through ongoing education and practice-oriented transfer strategies.

References

1. Statistisches Bundesamt (Destatis). Pflegestatistik 2021—Pflege im Rahmen der Pflegeversicherung—Deutschlandergebnisse. Wiesbaden: Statistisches Bundesamt; 2023. Available from: https://www.destatis.de/DE/Themen/Gesellschaft-Umwelt/Gesundheit/Pflege/_inhalt.html
2. Jacobs K, Kuhlmey A, Greß S, Klauber J, Schwinger A. Pflege-Report 2019: Mehr Personal in der Langzeitpflege—aber woher? Berlin: Springer; 2019. Available from: https://link.springer.com/chapter/10.1007/978-3-662-58935-9_17
3. Wolf-Ostermann K, Rothgang H. Digitale Technologien in der Pflege—Was können sie leisten? Bundesgesundheitsbl. 2024;67:324–31. https://doi.org/10.1007/s00103-024-03843-3.
4. IGES. Umfrage zum Technikeinsatz in Pflegeeinrichtungen (UTiP). Leipzig/Berlin; 2020.
5. Pflegepraxiszentrum Nürnberg. Implementierungsleitfaden: Eine praxisbezogene Arbeitshilfe zur Einführung technischer Innovationen in der Pflege. Nürnberg: PPZ Nürnberg; 2022. Available from: https://www.ppz-nuernberg.de/implementierungsleitfaden/
6. Krick T, Huter K, Domhoff D, Schmidt A, Rothgang H, Wolf-Ostermann K. Digital technology and nursing care: a scoping review on acceptance, effectiveness and efficiency studies of informal and formal care technologies. BMC Health Serv Res. 2019;19:400.
7. Greenhalgh T, Abimbola S. The NASSS framework—a synthesis of multiple theories of technology implementation. Stud Health Technol Inform. 2019;263:193–204. https://doi.org/10.3233/SHTI190123.
8. Frey CB, Osborne MA. The future of employment: how susceptible are jobs to computerisation? Oxford: Oxford Martin School, University of Oxford; 2013. Available from: https://www.oxfordmartin.ox.ac.uk/downloads/academic/The_Future_of_Employment.pdf
9. Greif S, Runde B, Seeberg I. Erfolge und Misserfolge beim Change Management. Göttingen: Hogrefe; 2004.
10. Stoumpos AI, Kitsios F, Talias MA. Digital transformation in healthcare: technology acceptance and its applications. Int J Environ Res Public Health. 2023;20:3407. https://doi.org/10.3390/ijerph20043407.
11. Kostka C. Change Management. Das Praxisbuch für Führungskräfte. München: Carl Hanser Verlag; 2016.
12. Westerman G, Bonnet D, McAfee A. Leading digital: turning technology into business transformation. Massachusetts: Harvard Business Press; 2014.
13. Ochoa-Urrego RL, Peña-Reyes JI. Digital maturity models: a systematic literature review. In: Digitalization: approaches, case studies, and tools for strategy, transformation and implementation, vol. 30; 2021. p. 70–85.

14. De Carolis A, Macchi M, Negri E, Terzi S. A maturity model for assessing the digital readiness of manufacturing companies. In: Advances in production management systems. The path to intelligent, collaborative and sustainable manufacturing. Springer; 2017. p. 13–20. https://doi.org/10.1007/978-3-319-66923-6_2.
15. Woods L, Dendere R, Eden R, Grantham B, Krivit J, Pearce A, et al. Perceived impact of digital health maturity on patient experience, population health, health care costs, and provider experience: mixed methods case study. J Med Internet Res. 2023;25:e45868.
16. World Health Organization (WHO). Monitoring the implementation of digital health: an overview of selected national and international methodologies. Copenhagen: WHO Regional Office for Europe; 2022.
17. Cresswell K, Jahn F, Silsand L, Woods L, Postema T, Logan M, et al. Assessing digital maturity of hospitals: viewpoint comparing national approaches in five countries. J Med Internet Res. 2025;27:e57858. https://doi.org/10.2196/57858.
18. Flott K, Callahan R, Darzi A, Mayer E. A patient-centered framework for evaluating digital maturity of health services: a systematic review. J Med Internet Res. 2016;18(4):e75. https://doi.org/10.2196/jmir.5047.
19. Duncan R, Eden R, Woods L, Wong I, Sullivan C. Synthesizing dimensions of digital maturity in hospitals: systematic review. J Med Internet Res. 2022;24(3):e32994. https://doi.org/10.2196/32994.
20. Healthcare Information and Management Systems Society (HIMSS). HIMSS adoption model suite. Chicago: HIMSS; 2023. Available from: https://www.himss.org
21. Organisation for Economic Co-operation and Development (OECD). Health at a glance 2023: OECD indicators. Paris: OECD Publishing; 2023. https://doi.org/10.1787/4dd50c09-en.
22. Geissler A, Quentin W, Busse R, Henschke C. DigitalRadar: Messung des Digitalisierungsgrades von Krankenhäusern in Deutschland. Berlin: IGES Institut; 2021.
23. Eymann T, Fürstenau D, Gersch M, et al. Das Reifegradmodell für den Öffentlichen Gesundheitsdienst—Ein Instrument zur Erfassung und Verbesserung des digitalen Reifegrades von deutschen Gesundheitsämtern. Bundesgesundheitsbl. 2023;66:136–42. https://doi.org/10.1007/s00103-022-03643-7.
24. Savic K, Büchner VA. Determinants of digital maturity models in healthcare sector and their relevance for long-term care facilities. Working Paper; 2025.
25. Seufert S. Digital Competences. Paper commissioned by the Swiss Science and Innovation Council (SSIC); 2017. Available from: https://wissenschaftsrat.ch/images/stories/pdf/en/Exploratory_study_3_2017_Excerpt_Digital_Competences_SSIC_EN.pdf
26. Brater M. Was sind „Kompetenzen" und wieso können sie für Pflegende wichtig sein? Pflege Gesellschaft. 2016;21(3):197–213.
27. Gesellschaft für Informatik. Leitlinien Pflege 4.0: Handlungsempfehlungen für die Entwicklung und den Erwerb digitaler Kompetenzen in Pflegeberufen. Bonn: GI; 2017. Available from: https://gi.de/fileadmin/GI/Hauptseite/Aktuelles/Aktionen/Pflege_4.0/GI_Leitlinien_Digitale_Kompetenzen_in_der_Pflege_2017-06-09_web.pdf
28. Seyda S, Placke B, Gensicke M. Digitale Kompetenzen in der Altenpflege im Vergleich zur Gesamtwirtschaft. IW-Report 7/2022. Köln: Institut der deutschen Wirtschaft; 2022. Available from: https://www.iwkoeln.de/fileadmin/user_upload/Studien/Report/PDF/2022/IW-Report_2022-07_digitale-kompetenzen-altenpflege.pdf
29. Havard M, Whistance M, Johns G, Drew S, Cusens C, Thomas S, et al. Defining digital nursing. Br J Nurs. 2024;33(2):72–7. https://doi.org/10.12968/bjon.2024.33.2.72.
30. Mainz A, Nitsche J, Weirauch V, Meister S. Measuring the digital competence of health professionals: scoping review. JMIR Med Educ. 2024;10:e55737. https://doi.org/10.2196/55737.
31. Bohnet-Joschko S, Mehulic L. Digital upskilling für die Pflege der Zukunft. PflegeZeitschrift. 2024;77(1):17–9. https://doi.org/10.1007/s41906-024-2591-2.
32. Rehe L-M, Heiland K, Zürn T, Mahler C. Digitale Kompetenzen von Praxisanleiter*innen. PflegeZeitschrift. 2024;77(3):39–42. https://doi.org/10.1007/s41906-024-2734-5.
33. Matusiewicz D, Werner JA. Future Skills in Medizin und Gesundheit: Menschen. Stärken. Kompetenzen. Berlin: medhochzwei; 2021.

34. Bundesministerium für Arbeit und Soziales (BMAS). Digitale Transformation in Pflegeeinrichtungen—Wie sich der Transformationsprozess gestalten lässt. Berlin: BMAS; 2024. Available from: https://www.bmas.de/SharedDocs/Downloads/DE/Publikationen/inqa-095-digitale-transformation-in-pflegeeinrichtungen-pdf.pdf
35. Kubek V, Velten S, Eierdanz F, Blaudszun-Lahm A. Digitalisierung in der Pflege—Zur Unterstützung einer besseren Arbeitsorganisation. Wiesbaden: Springer Vieweg; 2020. Available from: https://link.springer.com/book/10.1007/978-3-662-61372-6.
36. Santarsiero F, Schiuma G, Carlucci D, Helander N. Digital transformation in healthcare organisations: the role of innovation labs. Technovation. 2023;122:102640. https://doi.org/10.1016/j.technovation.2022.102640.
37. Tenggono E, Sudhartio L, Santoso A. Managing digital transformations: the intermediary function of digital readiness in facilitating strategic renewal within the healthcare industry. Cogent Bus Manag. 2024;11(1):2423276. https://doi.org/10.1080/23311975.2024.2423276.
38. Cheeseman SE. Are you prepared for the digital era? Neonatal Netw. 2011;30(4):263–6. https://doi.org/10.1891/0730-0832.30.4.263.

Part VII

Equity and Inclusion in the Digital Transformation of Healthcare

Responsible Use of AI: Ethical Considerations for Marginalized Groups

13

Stefanie Scholz

Referring back to previous chapters, AI has the potential to transform healthcare delivery by enhancing diagnostic accuracy, predicting health risks, optimizing resource allocation, and enabling personalized interventions. Yet, as with any transformative technology, its benefits and risks are not equally distributed. For marginalized groups—such as ethnic minorities, individuals with disabilities, people with low socio-economic status, the elderly, and populations in rural or underserved areas—the integration of AI into healthcare brings both opportunities for improved access and significant ethical challenges.

Ensuring that AI supports rather than undermines health equity requires an intentional focus on governance, inclusivity, and bias mitigation at every stage of the AI life cycle. This subchapter examines key ethical considerations for the responsible deployment of AI in healthcare with a focus on marginalized populations, structured around five core dimensions: data equity, algorithmic fairness, explainability and transparency, participation and co-design, and governance for accountability.

13.1 Data Equity: Representation and Quality

The reliability of any AI system depends on the quality and representativeness of its underlying data. When marginalized populations are absent or under-represented in training datasets, predictive models may perform poorly for these groups. For instance, diagnostic algorithms trained largely on majority-population data have been shown to misclassify conditions in patients with different skin tones or atypical symptom profiles [1].

S. Scholz (✉)
Faculty of Engineering, Ansbach University of Applied Sciences, Ansbach, Bayern, Germany
e-mail: stefanie.scholz@hs-ansbach.de

S. Scholz et al. (eds.), *Advancements in Digital Health and Care*,
https://doi.org/10.1007/978-3-032-16837-5_13

Data inequities can arise from several sources [2, 3]. Electronic health records (EHRs) may systematically contain less detailed clinical histories for individuals with inconsistent access to healthcare. Language barriers, cultural mistrust, and limited digital literacy can restrict participation in clinical trials or data collection initiatives. Moreover, historical patterns of exclusion and discriminatory practices have left notable gaps in longitudinal datasets.

Addressing these inequities requires targeted strategies. These may include purposeful data collection in under-represented communities, the careful use of synthetic data to increase diversity, and partnerships with trusted local organizations to improve completeness and accuracy [4]. Initiatives such as the European Health Data Space (EHDS) offer additional opportunities to strengthen diversity in datasets [5] (see Chap. 7 for a more detailed discussion).

13.2 Algorithmic Fairness: Detecting and Correcting Bias

Even when data is representative, algorithmic bias can arise from how models are designed, trained, and validated [6]. For example, risk prediction tools that incorporate variables correlated with socio-economic status—such as healthcare expenditure—can inadvertently deprioritize patients from lower-income backgrounds for advanced care interventions [7].

Ensuring fairness requires systematic bias assessment at multiple stages, drawing on measures such as disparate impact ratios or subgroup performance metrics. Tools such as *IBM's AI Fairness 360* and *Microsoft's Fairlearn* provide frameworks for evaluating and improving fairness. Validation should be conducted for diverse demographic, clinical, and geographic subgroups to confirm consistent performance [8]. Additionally, fairness-aware modelling techniques, such as re-weighting samples or introducing fairness constraints during model training, provide concrete means of mitigating the identified disparities [9].

Bias mitigation must be viewed as a continuous responsibility. Post-deployment monitoring is essential to identify changes in performance over time, particularly when these shifts disproportionately affect marginalized populations [10].

13.3 Explainability and Transparency: Building Trust in Marginalized Communities

Trust is a prerequisite for adoption, especially among communities with historical reasons for scepticism towards healthcare systems. Black-box AI models can cause distrust if patients or clinicians cannot understand how recommendations are made.

Explainability therefore carries both technical and ethical importance. Methods that make model behaviour more interpretable, such as feature attribution (e.g., SHAP, LIME), should be tailored for clinical use and explained in clear, accessible terms [11]. Transparency regarding data sources, decision-making processes, and system limitations should be an integral part of patient engagement, including disclosure of known biases [12].

Incorporating human-in-the-loop mechanisms allows clinicians to validate AI outputs while considering the patient's sociocultural context [13].

For marginalized groups, transparency should also address power asymmetries: making it clear who controls the AI system, how decisions can be appealed, and what recourse is available in case of harm.

13.4 Participation and Co-design Beyond the Dataset

Responsible AI is not solely about technical fixes—it also requires inclusive processes in which marginalized communities actively shape the tools intended to serve them [14].

Community-based participatory design, which brings together patient advocates, cultural mediators, and local healthcare providers in early development stages, can ensure that AI tools reflect the values and needs of the target population [15]. Equally important is capacity building, which equips community members with the knowledge and resources to engage critically with AI systems rather than remaining passive recipients [16].

Such participatory approaches can help ensure that AI systems do not inadvertently reinforce existing inequities or perpetuate stereotypes [17].

13.5 Governance, Regulation, and Accountability

Robust governance frameworks are necessary to protect marginalized groups from disproportionate risks. Under the EU AI Act, many healthcare-related AI applications are classified as "high-risk," requiring transparency, robust data and quality management systems, and human oversight [18, 19]. While this legislation offers a baseline, it must be operationalized with equity in mind. Equity-oriented governance could entail conducting impact assessments that explicitly examine differential effects on marginalized groups before deployment [20], ensuring that independent ethics review boards include representatives from the affected communities [21], and establishing clear mechanisms for liability and remediation when harm occurs [17].

Responsibility should be shared across all stakeholders—developers, healthcare providers, regulators, and funders—to ensure AI serves marginalized populations fairly [22].

13.6 Opportunities for Positive Impact

When designed and implemented responsibly, AI can help address longstanding barriers to care for marginalized groups. Remote diagnostic services can expand access to specialty care in rural and underserved regions [23, 24]. Language processing tools can support more inclusive, multilingual patient engagement [25].

Predictive analytics can identify at-risk patients earlier, enabling proactive interventions [26].

To realize these benefits, however, ethical safeguards must be integrated from the outset—not retrofitted after deployment.

The responsible use of AI in healthcare for marginalized groups is not a matter of optional ethical refinement—it is a core requirement for equitable digital transformation. Without careful attention to data equity, algorithmic fairness, transparency, participatory design, and governance, AI risks amplifying the very disparities it is capable of reducing.

For healthcare systems undergoing digital transformation, the ethical responsibility is twofold: to harness AI's potential for reducing inequities and to ensure that in doing so, no community is left behind. This requires sustained commitment, cross-sector collaboration, and continuous dialogue with those whose voices have too often been absent from the design and deployment of health innovations.

References

1. Cross JL, Choma MA, Onofrey JA. Bias in medical AI: implications for clinical decision-making. Cheungpasitporn W, editor. PLOS Digit Health. 2024;3(11):e0000651.
2. Chin MH, Afsar-Manesh N, Bierman AS, Chang C, Colón-Rodríguez CJ, Dullabh P, et al. Guiding principles to address the impact of algorithm bias on racial and ethnic disparities in health and health care. JAMA Netw Open. 2023;6(12):e2345050.
3. Gu T, Pan W, Yu J, Ji G, Meng X, Wang Y, et al. Mitigating bias in AI mortality predictions for minority populations: a transfer learning approach. BMC Med Inform Decis Mak. 2025;25(1):30.
4. Chen Z, Liang N, Zhang H, Li H, Yang Y, Zong X, et al. Harnessing the power of clinical decision support systems: challenges and opportunities. Open Heart. 2023;10(2):e002432.
5. Juhn YJ, Ryu E, Wi CI, King KS, Malik M, Romero-Brufau S, et al. Assessing socioeconomic bias in machine learning algorithms in health care: a case study of the HOUSES index. J Am Med Inform Assoc. 2022;29(7):1142–51.
6. Corbett-Davies S, Gaebler JD, Nilforoshan H, Shroff R, Goel S. The Measure and Mismeasure of Fairness. 2018 [cited 2025 Aug 12]; Available from: https://arxiv.org/abs/1808.00023.
7. Obermeyer Z, Powers B, Vogeli C, Mullainathan S. Dissecting racial bias in an algorithm used to manage the health of populations. Science. 2019;366(6464):447–53.
8. Subbaswamy A, Sahiner B, Petrick N, Pai V, Adams R, Diamond MC, et al. A data-driven framework for identifying patient subgroups on which an AI/machine learning model may underperform. npj Digit Med. 2024;7(1):334.
9. Ferrara C, Sellitto G, Ferrucci F, Palomba F, De Lucia A. Fairness-aware machine learning engineering: how far are we? Empir Software Eng. 2024;29(1):9.
10. Ueda D, Kakinuma T, Fujita S, Kamagata K, Fushimi Y, Ito R, et al. Fairness of artificial intelligence in healthcare: review and recommendations. Jpn J Radiol. 2024;42(1):3–15.
11. Ning Y, Liu M, Liu N. advancing ethical AI in healthcare through interpretability. Patterns. 2025;6(6):101290.
12. Frasca M, La Torre D, Pravettoni G, Cutica I. Explainable and interpretable artificial intelligence in medicine: a systematic bibliometric review. Discov Artif Intell. 2024;4(1):15.
13. Ennab M, Mcheick H. Enhancing interpretability and accuracy of AI models in healthcare: a comprehensive review on challenges and future directions. Front Robot AI. 2024;11:1444763.
14. Weiner EB, Dankwa-Mullan I, Nelson WA, Hassanpour S. Ethical challenges and evolving strategies in the integration of artificial intelligence into clinical practice. Kuo PC, editor. PLOS Digit Health. 2025;4(4):e0000810.

15. Hanna MG, Pantanowitz L, Jackson B, Palmer O, Visweswaran S, Pantanowitz J, et al. Ethical and bias considerations in artificial intelligence/machine learning. Mod Pathol. 2025;38(3):100686.
16. Nittas V, Chavez SJ, Daniore P. Current practice and expert perspectives on cultural adaptations of digital health interventions: qualitative study. JMIR Mhealth Uhealth. 2025;13:e59965.
17. Pham T. Ethical and legal considerations in healthcare AI: innovation and policy for safe and fair use. R Soc Open Sci. 2025;12(5):241873.
18. Busch F, Kather JN, Johner C, Moser M, Truhn D, Adams LC, et al. Navigating the European Union artificial intelligence act for healthcare. npj Digit Med. 2024;7(1):210.
19. Van Kolfschooten H, Van Oirschot J. The EU artificial intelligence act (2024): implications for healthcare. Health Policy. 2024;149:105152.
20. Gurevich E, El Hassan B, El Morr C. Equity within AI systems: what can health leaders expect? Healthc Manage Forum. 2023;36(2):119–24.
21. Dankwa-Mullan I. Health equity and ethical considerations in using artificial intelligence in public health and medicine. Prev Chronic Dis. 2024;21:240245.
22. Abràmoff MD, Tarver ME, Loyo-Berrios N, Trujillo S, Char D, Obermeyer Z, et al. Considerations for addressing bias in artificial intelligence for health equity. npj Digit Med. 2023;6(1):170.
23. Li DM, Parikh S, Costa A. A critical look into artificial intelligence and healthcare disparities. Front Artif Intell. 2025;8:1545869.
24. Okolo CT. Optimizing human-centered AI for healthcare in the Global South. Patterns. 2022;3(2):100421.
25. Chonde DB, Pourvaziri A, Williams J, McGowan J, Moskos M, Alvarez C, et al. RadTranslate: an artificial intelligence–powered intervention for urgent imaging to enhance care equity for patients with limited English proficiency during the COVID-19 pandemic. J Am Coll Radiol. 2021;18(7):1000–8.
26. Khanna NN, Maindarkar MA, Viswanathan V, Fernandes JFE, Paul S, Bhagawati M, et al. Economics of artificial intelligence in healthcare: diagnosis vs. treatment. Healthcare. 2022;10(12):2493.

Inclusive Digital Health in Higher Education: Accessibility, Well-Being, and Participation of Students with Disabilities

14

Marion Wüchner-Fuchs

14.1 Introduction

Digital transformation opens up new opportunities and flexibility but may reinforce existing inequalities if barriers remain in place. In particular, students with disabilities as well as those in special life situations (e.g., temporary physical or psychological impairments, multiple burdens from caregiving and parenting, linguistic and cultural adjustment challenges, high work-related pressures) find themselves navigating between new technological possibilities and persistent barriers. In the higher education context, digital health refers to the health-promoting, data-protection-compliant, and accessible design of digital teaching, counseling, and support services (e.g., e-mental health, tele-based counseling, digital exam accommodations). The aim of this chapter is to consolidate strategies for inclusive university development along the dimensions of accessibility, well-being, and participation in an implementation-oriented manner.

14.2 Inclusion: Normative and Educational Policy Foundations

Inclusion is both enshrined in human rights and mandated by educational policy. The UN Convention on the Rights of Persons with Disabilities (CRPD) defines equal access to education as an inalienable right, which also extends to digital learning environments. This creates a reform mandate for education systems and universities to systematically dismantle barriers—both analog and digital—and to shape participation within the framework of digital health in an equitable manner.

M. Wüchner-Fuchs (✉)
Department of Health, Education and Sciences, SRH University Heidelberg, Campus Fürth, Fürth, Germany
e-mail: marion.wuechner-fuchs@srh.de

S. Scholz et al. (eds.), *Advancements in Digital Health and Care*,
https://doi.org/10.1007/978-3-032-16837-5_14

14.2.1 Inclusive Education as a Human Right

Education is a fundamental human right to which all learners are entitled. It also represents a central means for the realization of other human rights: it enables liberation from poverty, promotes full participation in social life, and contributes to reducing exploitation. Against this backdrop, inclusion must be understood as a comprehensive reform process of the education system that requires profound changes at the levels of content, didactic approaches, institutional structures, and educational policies [1]. The goal is to remove barriers in favor of a participation-oriented educational experience for diverse learners.

14.2.2 Inclusive University as an Institutional Paradigm

An inclusive university ensures equal participation in education regardless of individual characteristics and embeds digital accessibility as well as health-promoting conditions. It carries a dual mandate: on the one hand, to qualify students for inclusive professional practice, and on the other, to provide an inclusive study environment itself.

Key design principles include:

(a) Accessible entry: Physical, digital, and didactic structures must be designed so that students with disabilities, chronic illnesses, or other limitations can learn without obstacles. Accessibility must be understood comprehensively (§ 4 Behindertengleichstellungsgesetz, BGG).[1]
(b) Social justice: Inclusion requires consideration of diverse social backgrounds and life situations. Universities are obliged to compensate for study-impeding inequalities through transparent admission procedures, targeted support instruments, and counseling structures. These include scholarship programs, support services for first-generation students, and measures to reconcile studies, employment, and family responsibilities.
(c) Didactic diversity: Teaching methods and examination formats should be aligned with the learning needs of students rather than primarily with the routines or preferences of lecturers. In an inclusive university, this means, for example, offering accessible examination formats, addressing heterogeneous prior experiences through differentiated assignments, and using activating teaching methods that engage students with and without disabilities equally.

[1] The German Disability Equality Act (Behindertengleichstellungsgesetz, BGG) is a federal law adopted in 2002 and subsequently amended, which aims to ensure equal rights and eliminate discrimination against persons with disabilities. It establishes the legal framework for accessibility in public services, buildings, transportation, and information technology. The Act obliges federal authorities to make their services, communication, and digital offerings accessible, thereby promoting equal participation in social life for people with disabilities.

Lecturers take on the role of moderators, systematically shaping the relationship between the learning environment and learning success.

(d) Non-discrimination: An inclusive university is a place where diversity is valued and where students feel accepted regardless of disability, gender, ethnic origin, religion, or sexual orientation.

(e) Structural support: Inclusion requires targeted measures such as financial assistance, counseling services, and the awareness-raising of both teachers and learners. University communication (internal and external) plays a decisive role in strengthening acceptance of and visibility for inclusion.

14.3 Accessibility: Digital Accessibility as a Prerequisite

Digital accessibility is a prerequisite for equal participation and an integral component of access to higher education in Germany. It is not an add-on but a quality criterion in teaching, counseling, and administration.

14.3.1 Technical and Didactic Dimensions

From a technical perspective, accessibility includes, among other things, screen reader compatibility, captioning/transcripts (including live captioning), semantically correct structuring of documents, and the use of accessible learning platforms. From a didactic perspective, it means designing teaching and examination formats as well as accommodations in such a way that different learning and communication needs are taken into account (e.g., flexible deadlines, alternative examinations, adaptive resources). Accessibility is therefore a pedagogical principle, not merely a technical standard.

14.3.2 Implementation Strategies

The implementation of digital accessibility requires a systematic, multidimensional strategy. Digital content is considered accessible if it can be used by all users, regardless of device, technical setup (browser, operating system), or existing impairments, without any loss of information [2]. The foundation of implementation lies in the principles of operability, perceivability, understandability, and robustness. These must, however, be translated into concrete procedures and testing mechanisms in order to ensure their effectiveness in everyday university practice. Examples include:

Interoperability: Open standards (e.g., LTI 1.3/OIDC, WebVTT/TTML, EPUB 3/ ISO/IEC 24751 "AccessForAll") connect teaching, counseling, and examination systems. In this way, an accessible application can be launched directly from the learning platform, and exam accommodations can be technically embedded—without disclosing sensitive diagnostic data.

Accessibility audits: Universities are already obliged under the Disability Equality Act (BGG) and the Ordinance on Barrier-Free Information Technology (BITV 2.0[2]) to make their digital services accessible. On June 28, 2025, the Accessibility Strengthening Act (BFSG[3]) additionally came into force, adapting certain digital products and services—including platforms used by universities—to European requirements (European Accessibility Act). Against this backdrop, learning platforms and websites are regularly reviewed and, if necessary, adapted according to international standards, particularly the Web Content Accessibility Guidelines (WCAG 2.1 or 2.2) (e.g., keyboard operability, semantics, screen reader compatibility). The same applies to examination and teaching materials, which must be created or converted in accessible formats in line with legal requirements, such as 3D models, Braille editions, or interactive digital resources. A key monitoring function is carried out by the supervisory bodies for accessibility established in the federal states: they check compliance with legal requirements, uncover shortcomings, and increase pressure for action on public institutions, including universities [3].

Qualification and awareness-raising of university staff: Staff members need specific knowledge about digital accessibility in order to implement it consistently in teaching, examinations, and services. Training should be practice-oriented, for example, in creating accessible teaching materials, using assistive technologies, or applying case studies for reasonable accommodations. In addition, guidelines and checklists support staff by making standards tangible and facilitating their transfer into daily work. Awareness-raising relates not only to technical aspects but also to disability as a broader topic: disability is often not addressed within university culture because it is perceived as "not belonging." As a result, disability-related needs are easily overlooked or misjudged. For example, the effects of a visual impairment vary depending on the type of eye condition—such as contrast sensitivity, depth of field, or visual field loss—which may require different forms of compensation. Qualification measures therefore contribute not only to skill development but also to fostering a culture of responsibility in which accessibility is understood as an integral part of quality assurance and inclusion.

14.3.3 Challenges

The implementation of digital accessibility is hampered by limited financial resources, a lack of expertise, and, at times, low institutional prioritization.

[2]The Ordinance on Barrier-Free Information Technology (Barrierefreie-Informationstechnik-Verordnung, BITV) is a German regulation that specifies accessibility requirements for public sector websites, mobile applications, and digital services, aligning them with the standards of the Web Content Accessibility Guidelines (WCAG).

[3]The Accessibility Strengthening Act (Barrierefreiheitsstärkungsgesetz, BFSG) is a German law that implements the European Accessibility Act. It defines binding accessibility requirements for certain products and services, including digital platforms used by universities, and came into effect in June 2025.

Nevertheless, it remains an indispensable prerequisite for equal education and participation. Inclusive university development is situated in the tension between dystopian scenarios—characterized by exclusion, selection mechanisms (keyword: elite education), and structural barriers—and utopian visions in which accessibility is not only consistently implemented but also regarded as a self-evident foundation of all academic and administrative practices. In this vision, diversity is understood as a central resource for innovation, justice, and social progress. How universities navigate these tensions will determine whether they reproduce existing inequalities or overcome them in a transformative way.

14.4 Well-Being: Digital Health and Psychosocial Dimensions

The Student Survey in Germany: best3 [4] shows that 15.9% of students report health-related impairments that make their studies more difficult—a significant increase compared to 2021 (11%). This development underscores the growing importance of psychosocial support and highlights the responsibility of universities to create supportive conditions for well-being in order to reduce dropout rates and ensure participation.

The digitalization of higher education not only changes learning and working processes but also affects the mental well-being of students. For students with disabilities or chronic illnesses in particular, issues of digital health are closely linked to inclusion. In this context, well-being becomes an educational policy and didactic guiding principle that takes into account both individual burdens and structural conditions.

14.4.1 Burdens and Opportunities

Digital formats open up diverse opportunities for students, such as flexible study times, participation in courses independent of location, and the use of assistive technologies. These factors can reduce barriers and facilitate the reconciliation of studies, therapy, and private life. At the same time, burdens arise, such as digital overload, constant availability, and increased cognitive demands due to complex learning platforms [5]. For students with disabilities, digital formats that are well-intentioned but poorly adapted to specific target groups often create multiple burdens: long online sessions can be overwhelming despite supportive tools such as captioning or sign language interpretation, while non-accessible PDFs create additional effort for visually impaired students.

These challenges are particularly severe for students with psychological disabilities, who at 65.2% represent the most common form of study-impairing condition. Schirl et al. [6] show that, for example, the symptoms of ADHD (prevalence in adulthood approx. 2.5% in Germany [7]) entail a wide range of challenges that continue beyond compulsory schooling into higher education. Such burdens affect not only learning and performance processes but also social interactions. Adolescents and young adults with psychological impairments generally report reduced well-being and simultaneously face difficulties in managing academic tasks [8].

14.4.2 Support Services

Institutionally anchored measures are required to promote digital well-being. These include, for example:

(a) awareness trainings on discrimination and accessibility for all members of the university (teaching staff, administration, students), which raise sensitivity for the psychosocial dimension of digital exclusion,
(b) psychosocial counseling services that take into account the particularities of digital study environments (e.g., stress caused by online examinations, uncertainty in handling assistive technologies) and,
(c) accessible e-mental health services or hybrid sports and relaxation programs [9].

Practical examples show that students with disabilities particularly benefit from low-threshold online counseling formats when these are consistently designed to be accessible and combined with individual support. E-mental health services are especially effective when they are WCAG-compliant, low-threshold (e.g., multilingual, Easy-to-Read language [10]), hybrid (online/offline), and when they are continuously evaluated using indicators such as usage rate, waiting time, and dropout rate. Self-help apps offering psychoeducation, exercises, and progress tracking have shown good to very good effects and should be part of university health management.

14.4.3 Prevention and Resilience

Universities can contribute to relief through protective concepts (e.g., clear rules on digital availability, time buffers for online examinations). Promoting resilience in higher education includes measures such as peer mentoring, reflection spaces for digital stress, or training programs for stress management [11]. It is also essential that universities do not address digital health as an individual problem of specific students but rather as a structural task. Digital learning and working environments must be designed in ways that support well-being instead of jeopardizing it.

14.5 Participation: Key to Sustainable Inclusion

The active involvement of students with disabilities is a prerequisite for needs-oriented measures, acceptance, and effectiveness. Co-design formats, sounding boards, and peer tutors support the sustainable anchoring of inclusive standards.

14.5.1 Co-governance and Binding Participation Rights

Participation is established as co-determination in decision-making processes, not merely as consultation. Universities guarantee students with disabilities permanent seats and voting rights in relevant committees (e.g., senate, examination boards, quality circles) and record this in official documents (e.g., Inclusion Action Plan). Accessible formats (sign language interpreting, Easy-to-Read language, hybrid participation, provision of appropriate background information) as well as compensation for expenses and allocated time budgets ensure the actual exercise of these rights. Example indicators: proportion of committees with reserved seats; number of decision-relevant documents with documented participation of affected students; budget allocated for accessibility and honoraria.

14.5.2 Participatory Monitoring, Evaluation, and Accountability

Quality objectives for accessibility, well-being, and academic success are defined jointly with students with disabilities and regularly evaluated. A public Inclusion Report compiles key figures, progress of measures, and corrective actions; an independent ombudsperson's office ensures complaint procedures and follow-up. Data collection is carried out in a diversity-sensitive manner (e.g., voluntary self-disclosure, multiple disability categories) and feeds back into planning and budgetary decisions. Example indicators: implementation rate of accessible teaching materials; processing time and quality of reasonable accommodations; dropout/transfer rates and student satisfaction.

14.6 Conclusion

Accessibility, well-being, and participation form a triad that is crucial for inclusive universities in the digital age. Universities that reliably embed these dimensions ensure equal opportunities and enhance the quality of academic education. The inclusive university is not solely oriented toward the removal of barriers but toward a fundamental cultural transformation: moving away from conformity and toward new patterns of academic practice. Inclusion thus becomes a future-oriented project that enables progress through alternative structures and ways of thinking. In this sense, inclusion can be understood as a process of a "new enlightenment"—a departure from self-imposed conformity toward a self-determined, equitable, and diversity-sensitive academic culture.

In parallel, inclusion also has a strategic dimension: with around 90,000 people with disabilities in Germany who, despite being qualified, are currently not studying, and approximately 12,000 more each year, inclusion also represents a strategic recruitment decision—with real growth potential for universities that institutionally secure accessibility, digital health, and participation.

Competing Interests The author declares no competing interests.

Ethics Approval Not applicable (no primary research involving humans or animals was conducted).

References

1. CRPD. Allgemeine Bemerkung Nr. 4/General comment No. 4. Document symbol: CRPD/C/GC/4. 2016.
2. Deitmer A, Möhring MM, Vilas-Boas da Silva JM. Status quo of digital accessibility in multinational enterprises—an exploratory study [Status quo der digitalen Barrierefreiheit in multinationalen Unternehmen – eine explorative Studie]. Int J Adv Intell Syst. 2024;17(1–2):112–21. Available from: https://www.thinkmind.org/articles/intsys_v17_n12_2024_10.pdf.
3. Deutsche Rentenversicherung Knappschaft-Bahn-See. Überwachungsstellen der Länder—Überwachungsstelle des Bundes für Barrierefreiheit von Informationstechnik (BVI). 2025. Available from: https://www.bfit-bund.de/DE/Kontakt/Ueberwachungsstellen-der-Laender/ueberwachungsstelle_laender_node.html.
4. Deutsches Zentrum für Hochschul- und Wissenschaftsforschung (DZHW). The Student Survey in Germany: best3. Studying with health impairments. 2023. Available from: https://www.dzhw.eu/pdf/ab_20/best3_exec_summary_en.pdf.
5. WHO. Global report on assistive technology. Geneva: World Health Organization; 2022.
6. Schirl J, Pessel N, Radoslavjevic M, Szép A, Chavanon M, Christiansen H, et al. Empirische Arbeit: Einflussfaktoren des Einsatzes evidenzbasierter Klassenrauminterventionen bei Schüler:innen mit ADHS: Perspektiven von Eltern, Kindern und Jugendlichen. Psychol Erzieh Unterr. 2024;71(4):212–28. https://doi.org/10.2378/peu2024.art22d.
7. AWMF. Aufmerksamkeitsdefizit-/Hyperaktivitätsstörung (ADHS) im Kindes-, Jugend- und Erwachsenenalter [AWMF-Registernummer 028_045]. 2017. Available from: https://www.dgppn.de/_Resources/Persistent/6f514fd31d75221054f1d880bda9637728e2b92d/Langfassung%20ADHS%20Leitlinie_080618.pdf.
8. Schellenberg C, Pfiffner M, Krauss A, Martin M, Georgi-Tscherry P. EIL—Enhanced Inclusive Learning Nachteilsausgleich und andere unterstützende Massnahmen auf der Sekundarstufe II. Schlussbericht. Zürich: HFH; 2021.
9. Voß-Nakkour S, Rustemeier L, Möhring M, Deitmer A, Grimminger S. Digitale Barrierefreiheit in der Bildung weiter denken: Innovative Impulse aus Praxis, Technik und Didaktik. 2023. https://doi.org/10.21248/gups.62773.
10. Inclusion Europe. Easy-to-read. 2025. Available from: https://www.inclusion-europe.eu/easy-to-read/.
11. Schneider DP. Lebenskompetenz- und Resilienzförderung im (digitalen) Lehr- und Lernsetting. Die Hochschullehre 2022;8. https://doi.org/10.3278/hsl2204w.

Part VIII

Innovative Development Paradigms for Healthcare Digitalization

15 Model-Driven Development and Low-Code Platforms in Healthcare Digitalization: Opportunities and Challenges

Jan Fritz Jikeli

Abbreviations

ABAC	Attribute-Based Access Control
API	Application Programming Interface
BPMN	Business Process Model and Notation
BSI	Bundesamt für Sicherheit in der Informationstechnik
CI/CD	Continuous Integration/Continuous Deployment
CIM	Computation-Independent Model
CMMN	Case Management Model and Notation
COTS	Commercial Off-The-Shelf
CPG	Clinical Practice Guidelines
DACH	Deutschland, Österreich, Schweiz
DICOM	Digital Imaging and Communications in Medicine
DMN	Decision Model and Notation
EHR	Electronic Health Record
ELGA	Elektronische Gesundheitsakte (Austria)
ePA	elektronische Patientenakte (Germany)
EPR/EPD	Electronic Patient Record (Switzerland)
FHIR	Fast Healthcare Interoperability Resources
GDPR	General Data Protection Regulation
HL7	Health Level Seven
IHE	Integrating the Healthcare Enterprise
ISO/IEC	International Organization for Standardization/International Electrotechnical Commission
KHZG	Krankenhauszukunftsgesetz
LCDP	Low Code Development Platform

J. F. Jikeli (✉)
mgm technology partners GmbH, Munich, Germany
e-mail: Jan.Jikeli@mgm-tp.com

S. Scholz et al. (eds.), *Advancements in Digital Health and Care*,
https://doi.org/10.1007/978-3-032-16837-5_15

LIS/RIS	Laboratory/Radiology Information System
MDA	Model Driven Architecture
MDSE	Model-Driven Software Engineering
MII	Medizininformatik-Initiative
NIS2	Network and Information Systems Directive 2
OAuth/OIDC	Open Authorization/OpenID Connect
OMG	Object Management Group
OWASP	Open Web Application Security Project
PIM/PSM	Platform-Independent/Platform-Specific Model
RBAC	Role-Based Access Control
SaaS	Software-as-a-Service
SDK	Software Development Kit
SNOMED CT	Systematized Nomenclature of Medicine—Clinical Terms
SSO	Single Sign-On
TI	Telematik-Infrastruktur
V&V	Verification and Validation

Trailer
Healthcare leaders face mounting pressure to modernize IT landscapes while upholding safety, compliance, and interoperability. Traditional software engineering often struggles to keep pace with regulatory change, integration demands, and the rapid evolution of digital health services. This chapter explores whether model-driven software engineering (MDSE) and low-code/no-code (LC/NC) platforms can provide a viable path forward. By combining formal models with rapid development capabilities, these approaches aim to shorten delivery cycles without compromising quality or regulatory assurance. We illustrate this potential through examples from the DACH region—including Germany's Hospital Future Act (Krankenhauszukunftsgesetz, KHZG), Austria's national electronic health record system (ELGA), and Switzerland's electronic patient record (EPR, Elektronisches Patientendossier)—and position LC/NC within the broader trend towards agentic software development. The discussion culminates in decision guidance for healthcare executives, offering criteria to evaluate LC/NC adoption in clinical environments.

15.1 Definitions and Core Principles

15.1.1 Definitions and Core Principles of MDSE

In regulated healthcare, model-driven software engineering (MDSE) is less about hand-coding and more about engineering durable systems that can evolve safely. Here, models function as operational knowledge interpretable by both humans and machines. They decouple clinical semantics from the underlying technology:

medical concepts can change at their own pace, while the technical stack can be renewed independently. This separation enables three recurring programme goals: reducing risk before go-live, supporting flexible adaptation to domain-specific and technical changes, and preserving the long-term value of applications.

In MDSE, models are not just documentation but the primary building blocks of a system. They describe the domain logic, behaviour, and architecture in a way that can be processed by machines. From these models, software is generated automatically through defined transformations and code generation [6]. The Object Management Group's Model-Driven Architecture (MDA) helps explain this process. It defines three kinds of models:

- Computation-Independent Models (CIM): focus only on clinical requirements and workflows, without any IT details.
- Platform-Independent Models (PIM): describe the system's structure and behaviour in general terms, still without tying it to a specific technology.
- Platform-Specific Models (PSM): adapt the PIM to a concrete technology or platform (e.g., Java, .NET, or a cloud service).

This layered approach makes it easier to move systems between technologies and to maintain them over time. Automated model-to-model and model-to-text transformations ensure consistency across layers. Domain-specific languages (DSLs) allow clinicians to describe medical rules and concepts in a formal, computable way. A common example would be a change in how laboratory values are interpreted. If the threshold for an abnormal blood glucose level is updated, this adjustment can be entered once in the model and then automatically applied across all generated parts of the system, ensuring consistency without manual re-coding. Another frequent case is medication dosage rules: if guidelines change the recommended maximum daily dose for a drug, the update is made once in the model and then carried through to all relevant software components, from prescribing modules to decision-support checks.

15.1.2 Definition and Characteristics of Low-Code/No-Code

Low-code/no-code (LC/NC) development reduces the amount of manual programming required to build software applications, enabling faster delivery through visual tools and automated generation. While both approaches minimize hand-coding, "low-code" platforms still allow limited scripting or configuration by developers, whereas "no-code" platforms are designed for users without any programming skills. LC/NC platforms apply model-driven principles in a practical way, offering visual modelling, reusable components, and automated generation of applications [4]. Their aim is to reduce repetitive project effort, enforce consistent standards, and enable faster delivery compared to traditional coding.

In enterprise settings, professional developers and domain experts collaborate using visual models, component libraries, and configuration rather than hand-coding most functionality. LC/NC tools that require no programming skills are often aimed at "citizen developers", but in healthcare the complexity of rules, integrations, and regulatory requirements usually demands enterprise-grade LC/NC rather than simple citizen-developer tools [1, 2, 8].

Key characteristics of LC/NC platforms include:

- Visual development: drag-and-drop editors for data, workflows, and user interfaces.
- Reusable assets: component and widget libraries that enforce consistency.
- Integration connectors: pre-built links to common systems (EHRs, LIS/RIS, billing, IAM).
- Policy as code: built-in access-control and compliance rules.
- Automation: pipelines for deployment, testing, and monitoring.

Healthcare contexts demand more than speed: platforms must expose artefacts transparently, align with standards such as HL7 Fast Healthcare Interoperability Resources (FHIR) and openEHR, and integrate into verification and validation (V&V) pipelines. As discussed in Sect. 15.2.3, a well-governed LC/NC programme blends clinical expertise with software-engineering discipline, avoiding unstructured citizen development and reducing vendor lock-in through openness and standards support.

15.2 The Relevance of MDSE

15.2.1 Benefits for Healthcare IT

MDSE offers several advantages for healthcare IT, but its limitations must also be acknowledged.

Benefits

MDSE promotes modularity and maintainability by decoupling clinical knowledge from technical implementation. This makes it easier to update medical logic without rewriting large parts of the system. It also strengthens compliance and traceability: models can be linked directly to standards and regulatory artefacts, supporting audits and life cycle processes ([10]; [20]). Furthermore, MDSE enables interoperability by encoding domain semantics in a structured, machine-interpretable way. When combined with standards such as HL7 FHIR (Fast Healthcare Interoperability Resources) or openEHR, this reduces bespoke interfaces and improves semantic consistency across systems. Finally, MDSE encourages early quality assurance. Because models are executable, prototypes and simulations can be validated before deployment, reducing risk and time-to-value [6]. Moreover, MDSE fosters long-term strategic benefits such as a more agile IT environment, increased innovation capacity, and improved patient outcomes through better digital tools.

Limitations

MDSE adoption requires specialized expertise in modelling languages and transformation pipelines. Without proper governance, models may fragment or drift from implementation, undermining their reliability. Tool ecosystems can also be vendor-specific, raising lock-in concerns and limiting portability though open-source frameworks such as Acceleo, Eclipse Sirius, and Capella offer alternatives that reduce dependency on proprietary solutions. Performance overhead is another risk: automatically generated artefacts may be less efficient than hand-crafted code in high-volume scenarios. Finally, organizational readiness is crucial. Beyond technical skills, MDSE adoption faces human and organizational challenges including resistance to change from established workflows, significant skill gaps among clinical and technical staff, and the need for new governance models to manage collaborative model development. Without addressing these factors, MDSE can become a bottleneck rather than an enabler.

In summary, MDSE brings strong benefits for compliance, adaptability, and interoperability in healthcare IT, but these gains depend on sustained governance, skills, and integration with established standards.

15.2.2 Modelling Artefacts and Languages in Healthcare

Model-driven software engineering (MDSE) in healthcare relies on a variety of modelling artefacts and languages. These artefacts serve as the bridge between clinical knowledge and technical implementation, ensuring that systems remain consistent, interoperable, and safe.

Clinical Content Models

A central example is openEHR, an international open standard for health data. Its key idea is to separate medical knowledge from technology. Clinical concepts such as blood pressure, allergies, or lab values are defined in reusable building blocks called archetypes. These archetypes describe in detail how a clinical concept is structured. For practical use, several archetypes are combined into templates, for example to represent a discharge letter or a diabetes assessment. This separation ensures that medical knowledge can be reused across projects, governed jointly by clinicians and IT experts, and validated automatically—while the underlying technical platform can evolve independently [14].

Process and Decision Models

Healthcare processes involve pathways, decision points, and case handling. Three notations from the Object Management Group (OMG) are widely applied:

- BPMN (Business Process Model and Notation): Describes end-to-end workflows such as patient admission or discharge [15].

- DMN (Decision Model and Notation): Captures decision logic using tables and rules, for example medication dosage based on patient parameters [17].
- CMMN (Case Management Model and Notation): Represents less structured, event-driven processes, such as handling complex oncology cases [16].

Together, these notations—often referred to as the Triple Crown—allow precise modelling of healthcare pathways and decisions, [5] making them executable and testable.

Computable Clinical Guidelines
Traditional clinical guidelines are written in natural language and thus ambiguous for machines. HL7's CPG-on-FHIR initiative transforms narrative guidelines into machine-readable artefacts, [12] such as recommendations, pathways, and quality measures. Using FHIR resources, these computable guidelines ensure that evidence-based practice can be directly embedded into clinical workflows and decision support tools.

Terminologies and Constraints
Safe interoperability requires unambiguous codes and robust data constraints:

- SNOMED CT provides a comprehensive clinical terminology for diagnoses, findings, and procedures.
- LOINC offers standard codes for laboratory tests and clinical measurements.
- RxNorm standardizes medication names and dosages for exchange across systems.

MDSE and LC/NC platforms can expose these terminologies as constraints in user interfaces and APIs, automatically validating data entries and preventing integration errors.

Safety Annotations
Safety requirements are increasingly attached directly to models. For example, potential hazards, mitigations, and risk controls—defined in standards such as ISO 14971—can be annotated within the models [18]. Automated linters and tests then verify that safety requirements are consistently implemented. NHS England's guidance further emphasizes embedding clinical safety checks throughout the life cycle.

15.2.3 Organizational Prerequisites and Governance

While Sect. 15.2.2 described the modelling artefacts and languages that provide the technical foundation, this subsection focuses on the organizational and governance prerequisites that ensure these models can be applied safely in healthcare. In short, strong governance closes the loop between conceptual models and their execution, preparing the ground for the practical tools discussed in Sect. 15.3.

Safety Leadership and Governance Structures

Clinical safety cannot be left to technology alone. Organizations must appoint Clinical Safety Officers with the authority and protected time to oversee safety throughout the life cycle. NHS standards DCB0129 and DCB0160 illustrate how to manage risks in development, deployment, and daily use, and these principles transfer well to model-driven pipelines. However, such standards are not yet systematically adopted across Europe, highlighting an important area for policy transfer and further research. Governance must therefore be dual in nature: combining clinical leadership with technical oversight.

Repository and Versioning Practices

Sustainable model-driven development depends on mature practices for storing and evolving models:

- Central repositories act as the single source of truth for all models.
- Semantic versioning makes it clear how each update changes meaning, not just structure.
- Peer review ensures that every change is checked by both technical and clinical experts before acceptance.

Verification, Validation, and Change Management

Verification and validation (V&V) should be integrated into pipelines, providing automated checks on safety, conformance, and performance. When changes are proposed, Change Advisory Boards should review model differences together with supporting test evidence, ensuring that updates do not compromise safety or interoperability.

Traceability and Design Controls

To remain auditable and compliant, every artefact should be linked along the chain from user need → requirement → model → test → deployment artefact. This traceability, emphasized in standards such as IEC 62304 [20] and ISO/IEC 25010 [19], makes it possible to show regulators and auditors exactly how requirements were implemented and verified.

15.3 Low-Code Platforms as Enablers of Digital Transformation

Building on the MDSE principles and governance prerequisites discussed in Sect. 15.2, the following subsections explore how LC/NC platforms operationalize these concepts to enable digital transformation.

15.3.1 Synergies with MDSE

Having defined LC/NC platforms, we now explore how they synergize with MDSE. LC/NC platforms can be seen as the practical implementation of MDSE: where MDSE provides the theoretical foundation—defining how models describe domains, behaviour, and architecture—LC/NC tools turn these ideas into usable platforms that clinicians and developers can apply directly.

Shared Principles
Both MDSE and LC/NC rely on models as first-class artefacts. In MDSE these are formal abstractions; in LC/NC they appear as visual workflows, forms, and data models. In both cases, automated transformations generate the technical artefacts needed for execution. This shared foundation makes the two approaches mutually reinforcing [6].

Benefits of Synergy
- Rapid feedback loops: Clinicians can interact with prototypes generated from models, ensuring requirements are captured early and accurately.
- Consistency across layers: Model compilers and interpreters align data, UI, and workflow layers, reducing translation errors between design and implementation.
- Governed adaptability: Controlled propagation of model changes supports fast adaptation to evolving clinical protocols and regulatory updates.
- Standards alignment: Combining MDSE rigour with LC/NC tooling helps encode FHIR, openEHR, and terminology bindings natively, lowering the cost of integration.

Healthcare Impact
Together, MDSE and LC/NC bridge the gap between abstract modelling and day-to-day clinical IT delivery. This synergy allows healthcare organizations to accelerate digitalization while still maintaining traceability, safety, and compliance.

15.3.2 Applications in Healthcare

With the foundational principles and synergies in mind, we now survey where LC/NC platforms are applied in healthcare. LC/NC platforms are increasingly used across healthcare, but their application varies by domain complexity and governance maturity.

Administrative and Operational Tools
LC/NC accelerate the digitization of routine workflows such as appointment scheduling, staff rostering, procurement, and patient communication portals. These applications benefit from visual modelling and pre-built connectors without exposing sensitive clinical logic.

Clinical Support and Patient-Facing Apps

In combination with model-driven principles, LC/NC can power patient portals [7], e-prescription flows, structured intake forms, and care-pathway support tools [3]. Visual models make it easier to update questionnaires or consent forms in line with regulatory change. For clinicians, rule-based decision support and order-entry workflows can be prototyped rapidly and validated against FHIR profiles.

Data Integration

Hospitals and research networks have begun experimenting with LC/NC for integration scenarios, as documented in early case studies ([1]; [8]): mapping HL7 v2 messages to FHIR resources, synchronizing laboratory or imaging results, or enabling secure patient-data exchange across institutions. Low-code's reusable connectors reduce bespoke coding, while governance guardrails ensure traceability and auditability.

Limits of Application

While LC/NC is effective for structured workflows, integration, and user-facing interfaces, it is less suitable for high-performance analytics, complex algorithms, or device-level software where safety and latency constraints demand specialized engineering.

In summary, LC/NC platforms provide rapid solutions in healthcare administration, patient engagement, and interoperability, provided that clinical safety, compliance, and life cycle governance are built in from the outset.

15.3.3 Landscape of Low-Code Platforms for Healthcare

This subsection examines different low-code platforms to show how MDSE principles work in practice. We can divide platforms into two main categories: general-purpose platforms that can be used across domains including healthcare (such as Mendix, OutSystems, Microsoft Power Apps, and A12) and purpose-built healthcare platforms that are designed specifically for clinical applications (such as Better Studio). This distinction helps organizations choose the right platform for their needs. While systematic comparisons of low-code platforms exist [13], healthcare-specific evaluations are still limited.

General-Purpose Platforms

General-purpose LC/NC platforms focus on rapid development, broad integration options, and large user communities [13]. However, they differ significantly in how well they support healthcare-specific requirements:

- Mendix provides visual development tools and a marketplace for reusable components. To integrate FHIR and HL7, users typically need custom connectors rather than built-in features.

- OutSystems offers high-performance development with strong DevOps support. Healthcare interoperability features (e.g., FHIR, DICOM) usually need to be developed by project teams. This increases the governance effort.
- Microsoft Power Apps works closely with the Microsoft ecosystem (Office 365, Teams, Dataverse). FHIR integration is available through Microsoft's broader healthcare cloud services but is not part of the core platform. Deployment is mainly cloud-based.
- A12 is a general-purpose platform that uses an MDSE-centred approach [13]. It supports healthcare standards including FHIR and HL7 v2, with governance features aligned with IEC 62304 and IEC 82304-1. Deployment options include on-premises, sovereign cloud, and hybrid setups, addressing digital sovereignty requirements in the DACH region ([25]; [26]).

Purpose-Built Healthcare Platforms

Purpose-built healthcare platforms are designed specifically for clinical:

- *Better Studio* targets healthcare application development with openEHR and FHIR at its core. It provides ready-made clinical data models and templates. This makes it faster to build standards-compliant applications. It focuses on interoperability and clinical data structures. However, comparative performance data and adoption numbers are not widely available.

Interpretation

The choice of platform depends on what an organization needs. Most general-purpose tools have mature ecosystems and enable rapid digitization. However, platforms like Mendix, OutSystems, and Power Apps often need significant customization for clinical-grade interoperability and regulatory compliance. A12 demonstrates that general-purpose platforms can also provide strong built-in support for healthcare standards and governance, reducing the customization effort. Purpose-built platforms like Better Studio go even further by designing the entire platform around clinical workflows from the start. However, they may have smaller user communities and less mature marketplaces than general-purpose alternatives.

In the DACH region, digital sovereignty is an important consideration. Hospitals and public authorities want control over data location, cloud dependencies, and compliance with national standards (e.g., BSI C5). Most general-purpose platforms rely on global cloud infrastructure. Platforms like A12 that offer sovereign or hybrid deployment options can meet these requirements through rigorous modelling, embedded governance, and standards alignment. Still, broader empirical validation would strengthen the evidence. This includes performance benchmarks, long-term adoption studies, and comparative safety assessments.

15.3.4 Interoperability and HL7 FHIR Integration

The Fast Healthcare Interoperability Resources (FHIR) standard has become the backbone of modern health IT integration. FHIR provides granular resources (e.g., Patient, Observation, Medication), RESTful APIs and extensibility mechanisms, making it well suited to LC/NC and model-driven platforms [11].

Opportunities
Mature LC/NC platforms can embed FHIR natively into their metamodels. Capabilities include:

- Resource modelling: visual editors that work directly with FHIR resources and profiles.
- Profile import: support for national implementation guides such as MII Core (Germany), US Core, or UK Core.
- Terminology services: binding to SNOMED CT, LOINC, and ICD, with validation at design and runtime.
- Conformance testing: automated checks against FHIR profiles and capability statements.
- Integration adapters: connectors for HL7 v2, DICOM, IHE profiles [35, 37], and bulk import/export scenarios.
- Subscriptions and eventing: support for push-based updates, crucial for clinical workflows such as new lab results or medication orders.

Challenges
Despite its modular design, FHIR adoption in practice is uneven. Local extensions, partial implementations, and immature servers can fragment interoperability. LC/NC platforms must therefore balance flexibility with rigorous validation to avoid "FHIR in name only" integrations. Performance also matters: large-scale FHIR transactions (bulk exports, analytics feeds) can strain generic runtimes if not optimized.

Regulatory Framework in Germany
In the DACH region—and particularly Germany—FHIR is not only a de facto standard but has been anchored in law and regulation:

- ISiK (Informationstechnische Systeme im Krankenhaus): Under § 371 and § 373 SGB V, hospitals must implement gematik's ISiK specifications, which mandate FHIR-based interfaces. Compliance is verified through defined test procedures and transition deadlines.
- ePA (elektronische Patientenakte): The nationwide electronic patient record, rolled out from January 2025, is built on FHIR and IHE standards. Healthcare providers are legally obliged to connect, with financial sanctions (e.g., reduced TI-Pauschale from mid-2025, further sanctions from 2027) if integration is delayed.

- gematik specifications: gematik publishes official FHIR implementation guides and packages (e.g., de.gematik.fhir.*) [30] that serve as binding reference artefacts for industry and providers. These define resources, profiles, and validation rules required for conformance.

DACH Perspective and Digital Sovereignty
In Germany, Austria, and Switzerland, FHIR is central to national initiatives such as KHZG, ELGA, and EPR. Low-code platforms that natively handle these profiles reduce custom integration work and strengthen compliance. At the same time, healthcare authorities increasingly demand deployment in sovereign or hybrid clouds to ensure that FHIR data flows remain under national and institutional control [25, 26].

In sum, FHIR offers a powerful foundation for interoperability, but only when LC/NC platforms treat it as a first-class concern with governance, conformance tooling, and sovereignty-aware deployment options. In Germany, compliance with ISiK and ePA regulations makes FHIR not only a technical best practice but a legal requirement for healthcare IT systems.

15.3.5 Performance and Scalability Considerations

Healthcare workloads are diverse, spiky, and safety-critical. LC/NC platforms must therefore be designed for both resilience and scalability.

Workload Patterns
Clinical systems often run long-lived workflows (e.g., care pathways, treatment authorizations) that require durable state and guaranteed execution. At the same time, integrations with Electronic Health Records (EHR), Laboratory Information Systems (LIS), or Radiology Information Systems (RIS) generate bursts of high-volume transactions, particularly during peak hours. LC/NC runtimes must manage idempotent retries, back-pressure on Application Programming Interfaces (APIs) and safe roll-back mechanisms to ensure clinical continuity.

Design for Scale
Key patterns include:

- Horizontal scaling at the API tier (Application Programming Interface tier) to handle large numbers of simultaneous requests.
- Durable state handling for workflow and decision engines.
- Asynchronous messaging for high-volume interfaces and background tasks.
- Model annotations for Service Level Agreements (SLAs), enabling automated verification of performance goals in pipelines.

Observability

Structured logs, metrics, and distributed traces provide transparency into runtime behaviour. Error budgets and Service Level Objectives (SLOs) can then be defined, monitored, and acted upon. This level of observability is critical for regulated healthcare, where performance failures can have patient-safety implications.

Optimization Strategies

Caching must balance speed with privacy and data freshness. Bulk FHIR exports should be queued during off-peak times. Mobile applications should support offline forms with conflict resolution and auditable synchronization. Data at rest and in transit must remain encrypted to meet GDPR and NIS2 requirements.

In summary, performance and scalability in healthcare LC/NC platforms are not optional technical extras but central safety requirements. Designing for predictable load, transparent observability, and secure optimization ensures that LC/NC solutions remain reliable even under the stress of real-world clinical operations.

15.3.6 Testing Strategies and Model-Based Testing

Testing in regulated healthcare cannot be an afterthought. LC/NC platforms must integrate testing into every stage of the life cycle, leveraging the strengths of model-driven approaches and adopting a shift-left testing mindset—bringing verification as early as possible into the design process.

Model-Based Test Generation

Models of workflows, decision logic, and access rules can be used to automatically derive test cases. For example, every path in a clinical workflow model can generate a test sequence, while decision tables can be transformed into unit tests for rule engines. This reduces manual effort and ensures coverage of edge cases.

Complex Rule Validation at Scale

Healthcare applications often encode hundreds of interdependent rules, from medication dosage checks to insurance authorization logic. Manual testing is infeasible at this scale. Automated test generation from models ensures that thousands of combinations can be validated systematically, reducing the risk of hidden conflicts or omissions.

Contract Testing for Interoperability

When integrating with Fast Healthcare Interoperability Resources (FHIR) servers or other standards-based systems, contract tests verify that both sides conform to agreed profiles and capability statements. Stub servers can be generated from FHIR profiles to test message exchange without relying on live systems.

Regression and Safety-Critical Tests
Regression suites ensure that safety-relevant behaviour remains stable as models evolve. For example, medication dosage rules encoded in models should always trigger the correct alerts in generated applications. Automated regression tests lock in this behaviour and flag deviations early.

Security and Access-Control Validation
Executable policies derived from Role-Based Access Control (RBAC) or Attribute-Based Access Control (ABAC) models can be tested systematically. For instance, regression tests can assert that only authorized roles may access sensitive datasets.

Governance Integration
Testing must be embedded into continuous integration and continuous deployment (CI/CD) pipelines. Visual diffs of models allow reviewers to understand changes and their potential impacts before release. Evidence from automated tests—functional, security, conformance, and rule validation at scale—should be bundled for audits and compliance verification [19].

In summary, model-based testing transforms verification from a late-stage activity into an integral part of the development cycle. By shifting testing left, automating large-scale rule validation, and embedding results into governance pipelines, healthcare organizations can improve coverage, compliance, and clinical safety assurance.

15.3.7 Data Modelling Patterns for Clinical Applications

Clinical applications must capture the complexity of care: it is longitudinal (patients are treated over years), episodic (care is organized around encounters or conditions), and role-based (different professionals contribute at different stages). Model-driven and LC/NC platforms can represent these aspects through well-established modelling patterns.

Patient Timeline
A patient record should provide a longitudinal timeline that links encounters, observations, procedures, and orders in chronological order. This makes it possible, for example, to track how blood pressure develops over time or to compare laboratory values across multiple hospital stays.

Episode Bundles
Clinical care often revolves around specific episodes, such as diabetes management or a hip replacement. Grouping all related data—diagnoses, medications, lab results, and follow-ups—into an episode bundle ensures consistency, easier retrieval, and more accurate quality reporting.

Task-Centric Records

Care delivery is not only about storing data but also about performing actions. Task-centric records link intent to action: for instance, a physician orders a medication, the nurse administers it, and both actions are linked in the record as a verifiable task chain.

Technical Expression

These patterns can be expressed as reusable model templates. They include guard-rails such as mandatory coding systems, allowed state transitions, provenance rules, and audit trails. Fast Healthcare Interoperability Resources (FHIR) entities—including Encounter, EpisodeOfCare, CarePlan, and Task—map directly to these templates. Implementation guides with explicit invariants and value-set bindings ensure that systems remain semantically consistent across institutions.

Anti-patterns to avoid:

- Over-denormalized forms: Putting all data into a single form leads to duplication and problems when values change. For example, storing a patient's address in multiple records creates inconsistencies when the patient moves.
- Monolithic mega-models: Combining unrelated domains (e.g., cardiology and billing) into one large model makes systems inflexible and hard to maintain. In practice, changing billing codes may require clinical workflow recertification, causing unnecessary delays.

A better approach is to design modular sub-models with clear contracts and independent life cycles. Warning signs of emerging anti-patterns include growing user complaints about redundant data entry and very high costs for simple changes. If legacy systems enforce awkward structures, an anti-corruption layer at the integration tier should protect the clarity of the core clinical models.

In summary, data modelling patterns make clinical complexity manageable. By structuring records into timelines, episodes, and task chains—and by avoiding anti-patterns—healthcare applications built on model-driven and low-code/no-code platforms can be extended, validated, and governed in a controlled manner while maintaining semantic consistency and regulatory compliance.

15.3.8 Accessibility and Clinical UX Considerations

Clinical environments are stressful, noisy, and often low-light. Software used in these settings must prioritize clarity, speed, and accessibility over decorative design. LC/NC platforms can support this by embedding accessibility and usability patterns directly into reusable components.

Core accessibility requirements. International standards such as the Web Content Accessibility Guidelines (WCAG 2.1), the EU Web Accessibility Directive (Directive 2016/2102), the German Barrierefreie-Informationstechnik-Verordnung (BITV 2.0), and EN 301549 define measurable requirements. These include sufficient colour contrast, scalable typography, keyboard navigation, predictable focus order, and assistive-technology support via Accessible Rich Internet Applications (ARIA) landmarks.

Design for clinicians under pressure. Interfaces should emphasize signal over noise: large hit targets, clear typography, keyboard shortcuts for rapid entry, and reliable error recovery. Inline validation with explanatory feedback helps clinicians understand rules instead of blocking workflows without context. Defaults should be safe and transparent.

Reusable design systems. LC/NC platforms can encode accessibility standards into design tokens, style guides, and component libraries. This ensures that every generated application inherits accessibility compliance without bespoke rework. Design systems should also support multilingual content, since patient-facing portals in the DACH region must provide legally required notices and consents in German and other national languages.

Life cycle integration. Accessibility must be planned and checked throughout the entire software life cycle, not only at the end. This means:

- Automated accessibility checks should run in the Continuous Integration/Continuous Deployment (CI/CD) pipelines, so that every new version of the software is automatically tested for issues such as colour contrast or keyboard navigation.
- Review gates should include a requirement that each release provides an accessibility statement and evidence of successful tests before it can go live.
- Training for developers, business analysts, and testers ensures that all roles understand and apply accessibility requirements consistently.

This approach makes accessibility a measurable quality attribute that is built in from the start rather than being added at the end.

15.4 Shared Models and Federated Interoperability in German-Speaking Countries

After covering the technical and conceptual foundations of model-driven and low-/no-code (LC/NC) development, this section looks at how these concepts are being implemented in the DACH region—Germany, Austria, and Switzerland. In all three countries, interoperability frameworks built on open, machine-readable models are increasingly replacing isolated, custom-built solutions. National initiatives now use standards like FHIR, CDA, or IHE profiles not just for data exchange, but as common models that can generate executable components. This unified approach creates a type of model-driven interoperability that speeds up development, reduces duplication, and strengthens digital sovereignty.

15.4.1 Germany: KHZG, ISiK and the Model-Driven Reform of Hospital IT

Germany's Hospital Future Act (Krankenhauszukunftsgesetz, KHZG) is investing several billion euros in modernizing hospital IT systems. The funding covers key areas such as patient portals, digital documentation, medication management, telemedicine, and IT security [28]. Since 2024, e-prescriptions have been mandatory for all patients with statutory health insurance [27], and from 2025 onwards, the electronic patient record (ePA) is being introduced nationwide using an opt-out model [28]. All these services are built on FHIR APIs defined in the ISiK specification series. Gematik's publicly available implementation guides, automated Titus test suites, and confirmation procedures transform the ISiK profiles into working interoperability models [29].

This means hospitals can develop or generate interfaces and data structures directly from these models instead of writing custom code from scratch. New model-driven toolchains—such as those using FHIR Shorthand (FSH/SUSHI) or open FHIR validators—enable developers to build compliant systems from the ground up. The Medical Informatics Initiative (MII) takes this approach further by applying it beyond patient care: A standardized FHIR-based core dataset and reusable consent models ensure that research and clinical data exchange follow the same structural principles [31]. This shows how shared models can speed up implementation and help organizations stay compliant even as regulations change.

15.4.2 Austria: ELGA and Model Governance Through ART-DÉCOR

Austria's Electronic Health Record "ELGA" is an established national EHR infrastructure that provides access to clinical documents, laboratory results, and medication lists. ELGA manages its CDA and emerging FHIR resources using ART-DECOR, an open-source platform that stores templates, value sets, and terminologies as version-controlled models [32]. Any change to a template—such as adding a new medication or observation structure—can be automatically applied to all dependent applications. Software built on these resources, whether using conventional development or LC/NC approaches, therefore achieves interoperability and consistency by design. In practice, this allows regional disease-management and e-medication projects to update their applications simply by synchronising with the latest model definitions rather than rewriting code.

15.4.3 Switzerland: EPD, IHE/CDA-CH, and the Shift Towards FHIR

Switzerland's Electronic Patient Record (Elektronisches Patientendossier, EPD) is currently undergoing legal and technical updates to increase participation and patient engagement [34]. The EPD architecture is based on IHE XDS for document exchange and uses national CDA-CH content profiles managed by eHealth Suisse [36]. All specifications are publicly available and tested at regular "Projectathons". Recent national initiatives are introducing FHIR-CH profiles for selected processes to complement the existing CDA-based workflows. Because these specifications are openly developed and can be tested automatically, hospitals can generate CDA or FHIR documents directly from structured data models—reducing the need for manual coding and ensuring that data exchange is multilingual and legally compliant.

15.4.4 Cross-Sector Learning: The OZG-Cloud and the A12 Platform Concept

A useful example from outside healthcare is Germany's OZG-Cloud initiative in public administration. Developed by Dataport, FITKO, and several federal states, the OZG-Cloud provides a federated, open-source cloud environment that standardizes how digital public services are implemented and shared across different Länder. Following the "Einer für alle (EfA)" principle—meaning "one for all"—modules for forms, workflows, and document exchange are built once and then deployed multiple times, while data ownership stays local.

Within this framework, the A12 platform developed by mgm technology partners demonstrates how model-driven principles work in practice. A12 separates domain logic, user interface definitions, and integration rules into declarative models, which are then used to automatically generate working services. In the OZG-Cloud context, this architecture ensures that EfA services develop consistently, can be tested against shared specifications, and can be redeployed across different IT infrastructures. A12 therefore shows how model-driven architectures can turn interoperability standards into maintainable, scalable solutions that avoid vendor lock-in.

15.4.5 Implications for Digital-Health Platforms and Sovereignty

The experiences from healthcare and public administration converge on a common principle: shared, standardized models enable sovereign digital ecosystems. If hospitals, insurers, and research institutions adopt open artefacts such as FHIR profiles, CDA templates, and IHE workflows as the basis for generation rather than integration, they can build software that is:

1. Faster to implement—artefacts can be generated from existing models.
2. Easier to maintain—updates propagate automatically through toolchains.
3. Compliant by design—validation against published profiles is automated.
4. Digitally sovereign—models and toolchains remain open, self-hostable and reusable across sectors.

Such an approach would transform current interoperability programmes into a federated health-cloud architecture similar in spirit to the OZG-Cloud. Instead of isolated projects, national health systems could rely on a common semantic and technical foundation—enabling innovation, ensuring conformance, and maintaining long-term autonomy.

15.5 Benefits and Challenges of Model-Driven LC/NC Solutions in Healthcare

Building on the shared-model approach described in Sect. 15.4, this section examines the benefits and limitations of model-driven and low-/no-code (LC/NC) development in healthcare. While early pilots mainly focused on rapid prototyping, current initiatives under KHZG, ELGA, EPD, and MII show that LC/NC approaches can deliver FHIR- and IHE-compliant services at scale—as long as governance, security, and sovereignty requirements are built in from the start. The discussion covers four areas: technical, organisational, regulatory, and strategic.

15.5.1 Technical Considerations

Model-driven LC/NC pipelines can significantly reduce development time by automatically generating components—forms, APIs, validation logic—from common FHIR or CDA profiles. However, healthcare environments place exceptional demands on performance, scalability, and safety. Automatically generated components may need further optimization to handle high-volume FHIR transactions or imaging workloads.

Security is particularly critical: the OWASP LC/NC Top 10 highlights common vulnerabilities such as weak authentication, excessive permissions, and data leakage [22]. To address these risks, generated systems must include single sign-on (SSO), fine-grained role-based and attribute-based access control (RBAC/ABAC), encryption for data in transit and at rest, and continuous monitoring [23, 25, 26].

Model based testing is equally important: quality gates should validate clinical rules and access policies against shared FHIR or CDA models [19]. Only when model generation, validation, and testing work together in a continuous cycle can healthcare systems combine clinical safety and performance with development agility.

15.5.2 Organizational Considerations

While LC/NC environments make development more accessible, they can also lead to shadow IT if governance is insufficient. To prevent this, hospitals are establishing Centres of Excellence (CoEs) to maintain templates, ensure that verified components are reused, and control releases. Training is essential: clinicians, modellers, and IT staff need to learn how to co-develop components—interpreting visual workflows and understanding what the models mean.

Effective change management depends on transparent versioning, documented test results, and regular user feedback. Metrics such as task-completion time, incident reduction, or profile-validation rates can demonstrate improvement [1, 9]. Ultimately, LC/NC adoption only succeeds when organizations treat modelling as a shared, traceable discipline rather than an ad-hoc configuration activity.

15.5.3 Regulatory and Compliance Considerations

Health software regulation in Europe requires documented compliance with multiple frameworks. The GDPR (Article 9) governs the processing of health data, while medical device software must follow IEC 62304 and IEC 82304-1 [21]. National laws add additional requirements:

- In Germany, KHZG and ISiK require certified FHIR interfaces [28, 29].
- In Austria, ELGA and e-Medikation are defined by federal law [32].
- In Switzerland, the EPD law specifies CDA-CH and IHE compliance (BAG 2025; [33]).

LC/NC platforms operating in these environments must therefore provide audit trails, automated compliance validation, and policy-as-code mechanisms that enforce access rules directly at the model level. Model-driven components support this compliance: when a regulatory template or FHIR profile changes, all dependent modules can be automatically regenerated with updated validation logic—turning compliance into a repeatable engineering process.

15.5.4 Strategic Considerations and Digital Sovereignty

Strategic debates increasingly focus on digital sovereignty—the ability to deploy, audit, and develop software without external dependencies [24]. Proprietary LC/NC runtimes or closed modelling languages create vendor lock-in, which undermines long-term independence. The DACH region's public sector experience provides a useful model: the OZG-Cloud operates as an open, federated environment where model-driven components are shared nationwide (FITKO 2023; Dataport 2025). Within that ecosystem, the A12 platform shows how declarative, model-based generation can speed up service delivery while remaining compatible with open standards.

Applied to healthcare, the same principle supports sovereign health-cloud architectures: shared FHIR or CDA models, open toolchains (ART-DECOR, FSH/SUSHI, Camunda, Keycloak, Blaze FHIR), and federated governance ensure portability and independence from any single vendor. Key criteria for selecting platforms therefore include:

1. Openness—use of standard APIs and exportable models.
2. Portability—ability to deploy across sovereign or hybrid clouds.
3. Alignment—compatibility with ISiK, ELGA, and EPD profiles.
4. Sustainability—transparent roadmap and long-term vendor or community commitment.
5. Governance maturity—established safety, testing, and version-control policies.

Balancing short-term speed with long-term control is essential to avoid repeating past cycles of fragmentation and vendor lock-in.

Summary
Model-driven LC/NC development can deliver substantial benefits—speed, adaptability, and built-in compliance—when combined with strong governance and open standards. Beyond immediate efficiency gains, organizations can achieve long-term strategic benefits such as a more agile IT environment, increased innovation capacity, and improved patient outcomes through better digital tools. However, the challenges are equally multifaceted: technical performance, organizational discipline, regulatory compliance, and strategic sovereignty must all be managed together. The lesson from both DACH healthcare and the OZG-Cloud/A12 experience is that agility and sovereignty are not competing goals but complementary outcomes of a federated, model-based architecture. Only by treating shared models as primary, auditable components can healthcare achieve sustainable, sovereign digital transformation.

15.6 Conclusion and Outlook

The preceding analysis has demonstrated that MDSE and LC/NC development can transform the digital foundations of healthcare when they are anchored in governance, interoperability, and open standards. The chapter began by outlining how models as first-class artefacts enable traceability and semantic alignment across complex clinical environments. It then connected these theoretical principles with the practical architectures and national frameworks introduced in Sects. 15.4 and 15.5, showing that shared interoperability models—FHIR, CDA and IHE—constitute not only technical standards but a new methodological layer for federated innovation.

The evidence from Germany, Austria and Switzerland indicates that MDSE and LC/NC methods, when combined with open implementation guides, can substantially reduce redundancy and accelerate deployment. Germany's ISiK and KHZG programmes, Austria's ELGA ecosystem, and Switzerland's EPD framework illustrate how interoperability models act as living artefacts whose evolution can be governed collectively. The parallel developments in public administration, particularly the OZG-Cloud and the A12 platform, show that declarative, model-based generation can also operate at national scale while preserving local data control (FITKO 2023; Dataport 2025; mgm 2023). Together, these experiences suggest that shared modelling infrastructures could evolve into a "federated health cloud", combining reuse, transparency, and digital sovereignty.

From a technical and organizational perspective, the advantages of model-driven LC/NC development lie in reproducibility and adaptability. Automatically generated artefacts are consistent by construction, and updates to the underlying models propagate through all dependent modules. Yet these benefits depend on disciplined governance, continuous validation, and protection against security and performance risks. As highlighted in Sect. 15.5, the Low-Code/No-Code Top 10 (2023) underscores vulnerabilities such as weak authentication and excessive privileges, which must be mitigated by integrated identity management, encryption, and monitoring [25, 26]. Organizationally, new roles—clinical modellers, data stewards, and safety officers—become crucial to maintain the link between domain expertise and technical automation [1, 9].

Beyond these operational concerns, the most profound opportunity may lie in what can be termed agentic modelling with artificial intelligence [39]. Emerging research explores how AI agents can participate directly in the model-driven life cycle—reading regulatory texts, suggesting model updates, generating test cases, and detecting inconsistencies across FHIR profiles or policy rules [38]. Unlike traditional code-generation approaches, agentic modelling focuses on the meta-level: the AI operates on models rather than source code, producing explainable artefacts that remain subject to human review. This paradigm could transform how healthcare systems adapt to regulatory or clinical change. For instance, when new data-protection clauses or interoperability requirements are issued, agents could extract the relevant constraints, propose model adjustments, and run validation scenarios automatically. Human experts would then verify and approve these changes, maintaining the legal and clinical accountability of the system.

Such a collaboration between human governance and machine reasoning promises a new form of continuous compliance by design. Instead of periodic manual audits, regulatory assurance could become a dynamic process in which models, agents, and validation tools interact. In the longer term, a network of federated model repositories—synchronized through shared ontologies and policy rules—could allow European healthcare institutions to co-evolve their digital infrastructures while remaining locally sovereign. The combination of MDSE rigour, LC/NC accessibility, and agentic automation thus offers a pathway to faster yet safer transformation, bridging the gap between regulatory complexity and practical implementation.

Nevertheless, the approach requires careful safeguards. Agentic systems must remain transparent, traceable, and bounded by explicit governance frameworks. They should record every inference, justify modifications, and restrict autonomous actions to the modelling layer. Ethical oversight and human-in-the-loop validation are indispensable to ensure that AI-assisted updates do not introduce latent bias or compromise clinical safety. If these conditions are met, agentic modelling could redefine software evolution in regulated environments—not by replacing human developers, but by amplifying their ability to reason across the expanding web of standards, terminologies, and policies.

The combination of MDSE, LC/NC platforms, and agentic AI opens several important research areas. Key questions include how to formalize healthcare models so that both developers and AI agents can reliably work with them, and how model-driven architectures can scale across federated systems while maintaining consistency when many institutions use local variations of shared models.

Technical priorities focus on hybrid approaches that combine generated components with hand-written code while keeping everything traceable and testable. Research is also needed on optimizing performance for high-volume clinical workloads and integrating model-driven methods with microservice architectures.

Agentic modelling raises questions about how AI and humans should work together in regulated environments. How should agents propose and document model changes? What verification methods ensure that AI-generated modifications maintain clinical safety? How can we keep agent systems explainable and auditable?

Other critical areas include governance (how Centres of Excellence manage model libraries and train clinical staff), security (privacy-preserving model sharing and audit mechanisms), and evaluation (measuring quality and safety compared to traditional development). Cross-sector learning from finance, public administration, and manufacturing could reveal useful patterns. Addressing these questions will be essential to realize the full potential of MDSE-centred LC/NC ecosystems in healthcare.

The implications reach beyond healthcare. The interplay between model-driven design, LC/NC toolchains, and AI-assisted reasoning may represent a general paradigm for the public sector: one in which shared, interpretable models mediate between legislation and execution. Ongoing research in federated FHIR tooling [11, 31], policy-as-code frameworks [23, 26], and hybrid edge-cloud architectures will further define how such ecosystems operate.

Although the empirical evidence in this chapter is primarily drawn from the DACH region, the underlying principle is broadly transferable: semantic interoperability and governance automation are not regional peculiarities but structural requirements of any data-intensive domain. Implementing these ideas will require gradual institutional learning, integration with identity and access management, automated testing, and careful piloting. The central lesson is conceptual rather than procedural: sustainable digital transformation emerges when models, automation, and governance are treated as interdependent elements of a single socio-technical system.

In conclusion, model-driven and LC/NC development, strengthened by AI-based agentic modelling, provides a coherent strategy for reconciling speed with accountability in digital health. It transforms software engineering from a craft into a continuously verifiable process of knowledge representation and execution. When supported by open standards, sovereign infrastructure and transparent oversight, this approach can deliver a healthcare IT landscape that is not only faster and more adaptive, but also safer, more explainable, and fundamentally more human-centred.

Acknowledgements The author acknowledges the use of AI assistance (ChatGPT) in preparing this chapter, in line with Springer's guidelines on AI in academic publishing.

References

1. Ajimati MO, Carroll N, Maher M. Adoption of low-code and no-code development: a systematic literature review and future research agenda. J Syst Softw. 2025;222:112300. https://doi.org/10.1016/j.jss.2024.112300.
2. Al Alamin MA, Ghani SA, Ahmad R. Developer discussion topics on the adoption and barriers of low-code software development: an empirical study of stack overflow posts. Empir Softw Eng. 2022;27:1–34. https://doi.org/10.1007/s10664-022-10244-0.
3. Alomar D, et al. Patient access to electronic health records: a systematic review. J Med Internet Res. 2024;26(1):e56473. https://doi.org/10.2196/56473.
4. Bock AC, Frank U. Low-code platform development. Bus Inf Syst Eng. 2021;63:733–40. https://doi.org/10.1007/s12599-021-00726-8.
5. Bogale B, Vesinurm M, et al. Visual modelling languages in patient pathways: a scoping review. Interact J Med Res. 2024;13:e55865. https://doi.org/10.2196/55865.
6. Brambilla M, Cabot J, Wimmer M. Model-driven software engineering in practice. 3rd ed. Cham: Springer; 2022. https://doi.org/10.1007/978-3-031-02546-4_4.
7. Carini E, Villani M, et al. Impact of patient portals on healthcare outcomes: updated systematic review. J Med Internet Res. 2021;23(9):e26189. https://doi.org/10.2196/26189.
8. Martinez E, Pfister L. Benefits and limitations of low-code in construction. Autom Constr. 2023;150:104921. https://doi.org/10.1016/j.autcon.2023.104909.
9. Rokis K, Bravos G, Lapatas V. Exploring low-code development. Complex Syst Inform Model Q. 2023;36:57–85. https://doi.org/10.7250/csimq.2023-36.04.
10. Walderhaug S, Mikalsen M, Schabetsberger T. Model-driven traceability in healthcare information systems. Int J Med Inform. 2010;79(10):e333–41. https://pubmed.ncbi.nlm.nih.gov/20841686/.
11. HL7 International. FHIR Release 4.0.1 Specification. 2019. https://hl7.org/FHIR/R4/.
12. HL7 International. Clinical guidelines (CPG-on-FHIR) Implementation Guide v2.0.0. 2023. https://build.fhir.org/ig/HL7/cqf-recommendations/.
13. Kirchhof JC, Jansen N, Rumpe B, Wortmann A. Navigating the low-code landscape: a comparison of development platforms. In: Proceedings of MODELS, workshop LowCode. ACM/IEEE; 2023. p. 854–62.
14. openEHR International. Archetype technology overview. 2022. https://specifications.openehr.org/releases/AM/development/Overview.html.
15. OMG. Business Process Model and Notation (BPMN), Version 2.0.2. 2013. https://www.omg.org/spec/BPMN/2.0.2/.
16. OMG. Case Management Model and Notation (CMMN), Version 1.1. 2016. https://www.omg.org/spec/CMMN/1.1/.
17. OMG. Decision Model and Notation (DMN), Version 1.4. 2021. https://www.omg.org/spec/DMN/1.4/.
18. ISO. ISO 14971:2019—medical devices—application of risk management to medical devices. Geneva: ISO; 2019.
19. ISO/IEC. ISO/IEC 25010:2023—systems and software quality model. Geneva: ISO; 2023.
20. IEC. IEC 62304:2006—medical device software—software life cycle processes. Geneva: IEC; 2006.
21. IEC. IEC 82304–1:2016—health software—part 1: general requirements for product safety. Geneva: IEC; 2016.
22. OWASP. Low-Code/No-Code Top 10 Security Risks. 2025. https://owasp.org/www-project-top-10-low-code-no-code-security-risks/.

23. GDPR. Regulation (EU) 2016/679 (general data protection regulation). Off J Eur Union. 2016. https://eur-lex.europa.eu/eli/reg/2016/679/oj.
24. EU. Regulation (EU) 2023/2854 of the European Parliament and of the Council (Data Act). Off J Eur Union. 2023. https://eur-lex.europa.eu/legal-content/EN/TXT/?uri=CELEX%3A32023R2854.
25. BSI. Cloud computing compliance criteria catalogue (C5:2020). Bundesamt für Sicherheit in der Informationstechnik. 2020. https://www.bsi.bund.de/c5.
26. ENISA. NIS2 technical implementation guidance. European Union Agency for Cybersecurity. 2025. https://www.enisa.europa.eu/publications/nis2-technical-implementation-guidance.
27. BMG. E-Rezept: Einführung und Anwendung. Berlin: Bundesministerium für Gesundheit; 2024. https://www.bundesgesundheitsministerium.de/e-rezept
28. BMG. ePA für alle / Krankenhauszukunftsgesetz. Bundesministerium für Gesundheit, Berlin. 2025. https://www.bundesgesundheitsministerium.de/krankenhauszukunftsgesetz.html.
29. gematik. Elektronische Patientenakte (ePA). 2025. https://fachportal.gematik.de/anwendungen/elektronische-patientenakte-fuer-alle.
30. gematik. Telematikinfrastruktur und E-Rezept-Spezifikationen. 2024–2025. https://fachportal.gematik.de/.
31. Medizininformatik-Initiative. Kerndatensatz. 2025. https://www.medizininformatik-initiative.de/de/mii-kerndatensatz-neue-versionen-veroeffentlicht.
32. ELGA GmbH. About ELGA. 2025. https://www.elga.gv.at/.
33. eHealth Suisse. Elektronisches Patientendossier (EPD). 2025. https://www.e-health-suisse.ch/.
34. Schweizer Parlament. Revision des EPD-Gesetzes. 2025. https://www.parlament.ch/.
35. IHE Europe. Leveraging IHE methodology for the EHDS (White Paper). 2025. https://www.ihe-europe.net/.
36. IHE. Profiles for EPR and ELGA integration. 2023–2025. https://profiles.ihe.net/.
37. DICOM Standards Committee. DICOM PS3.1—introduction and overview. NEMA. 2025. https://www.dicomstandard.org/.
38. Li X, Huang L, et al. Enabling telemedicine: a scoping review. J Med Internet Res. 2025;27:e65932. https://doi.org/10.2196/65932.
39. Cabot J. Vibe modeling: challenges and opportunities. arXiv preprint arXiv:2507.23120.2025. https://arxiv.org/abs/2507.23120.

Part IX

Large Language Models and Conversational AI in Healthcare

Leveraging Large Language Models in Healthcare: From Speech Documentation to Conversational Agents

16

Christian Winkler

16.1 The Rise of LLMs in Healthcare

16.1.1 Introduction

Large language models (LLMs) have moved rapidly from research demos to pilots and early deployments across clinical workflows, patient communication, and biomedical research. Clinically oriented LLMs like Med-PaLM [19] or Med-Gemini [10] now achieve exam-level performance on many benchmark tasks, and multiple randomized and observational studies show that they can improve clinician productivity and decision-support—but important failure modes (hallucinations, bias, privacy, and regulatory uncertainty) remain [9]. Regulatory agencies are responding with lifecycle and marketing-submission guidance these systems and call them "AI as a medical device" [13]. Healthcare organizations should adopt LLMs cautiously, using retrieval-augmented approaches [2, 47], human-in-the-loop workflows, and rigorous local validation before clinical use [11].

16.1.2 LLMs

LLMs are large neural networks using the transformer architecture [50]. They are trained on massive amounts of text; sometimes images and other types of content is also used. After training, these models can generate, summarize, translate, and reason about language. So-called fine-tuning [41] is extremely effective and allows adapting the models to specific domains. Using retrieval augmented generation [2]

C. Winkler (✉)
Faculty of Business Administration, Technical University of Applied Sciences Nürnberg Georg Simon Ohm, Nürnberg, Germany
e-mail: christian.winkler@th-nuernberg.de

S. Scholz et al. (eds.), *Advancements in Digital Health and Care*,
https://doi.org/10.1007/978-3-032-16837-5_16

Table 16.1 Timeline of LLM usage in healthcare

2020	Release of GPT-3 [6], shows potential for medical Q&A, sparking initial experiments in healthcare text generation
Nov 2022	Release of ChatGPT [40] sparks the gen AI boom
2022–2023	LLMs like the GPT family [6] and PaLM [36] are tested for medical Q&A; first results look convincing, but problems like hallucinations remain
2023–2024	Medical fine-tuning and specialized models like Med-PaLM [19] and Med-PaLM-2 [47] show improved benchmark scores and excel in clinical evaluations
2024–2025	Randomized trials and implementation studies exploring LLMs for drafting patient messages [16], decision support, and diagnostic assistance; regulators (FDA) publish lifecycle and marketing-submission recommendations for AI/ML devices [21]

restricts the knowledge base to a set of expert documents and makes hallucinations much less likely while allowing more frequently updated content.

16.1.3 LLMs in Healthcare

In healthcare applications, several precautions need to be taken. Safety-critical decisions, privacy (personal health information, PHI), heterogeneous data (EHR notes, images, labs), and legal/regulatory obligations amplify both potential benefits and risks. Review articles analyze the clinical tasks where LLMs show promise. Among these are documentation, triage, coding, summarization, and clinical decision support [2, 29].

With a slow beginning, the adoption speed of LLMs in healthcare has increased in the last few years (see Table 16.1).

16.1.4 Examples of Existing LLM-Based Healthcare Applications

Documentation and inbox triage are used for drafting clinic letters, creating replies in the patient portal [16], and coding suggestions. Improvements have been shown in clinician efficiency in multiple QI (quality improvement) studies [23]. Clinical decision support uses LLMs to get and check differential diagnoses [11], guideline retrieval, and treatment suggestions when integrated as assistive tools (not autonomous). Clinical evaluations show potential but mixed reliability [18]. Patient engagement and education—introduces scalable, personalized explanations of conditions and meds, with risk of inaccuracies if not verified [49].

Multimodal clinical tasks use models that combine images and text (e.g., radiology, dermatology) that are emerging as successors for Med-Gemini and Med-PaLM [10, 19]. LLMs are also used for biomedical research and summarization; researchers have performed a literature study, generated hypotheses, and drafted protocols. The focus was on data extraction from unstructured content [2].

16.1.5 Measuring Success

Although not all these solutions work out of the box, a lot of success can already be observed. Med-PaLM [19] and Med-PaLM-2 show large gains on medical QA and exam-style benchmarks; Med-PaLM 2 reported large performance increases across MedQA/MedMCQA/PubMedQA [47]. Additionally, randomized and observational studies indicate LLMs can aid diagnostic reasoning and administrative tasks, but results vary with prompt design, grounding (retrieval), and clinician supervision. Some trials found improvements in speed and/or accuracy of diagnostics; others flag overreliance (physicians believe everything the LLM proposes) or error propagation, i.e., erroneous training information influences LLM predictions [11, 18].

The field is evolving rapidly; systematic review articles map promising roles but emphasize the lack of large-scale, multisite clinical outcome studies and standardized evaluation frameworks [9, 29].

16.1.6 Risks Using LLMs in Healthcare

No new technology goes without risks; some of those associated with LLMs can be challenging. LLMs can produce plausible but incorrect statements called hallucinations. This is especially dangerous in clinical advice. Later chapters shed some light on possible mitigation like retrieval augmentation, citations, human verification, or conservative prompting [2]. Another problem is bias and fairness as training data biases can amplify disparities. To cure that, domain-specific fine-tuning and specially curated audit datasets can be used for verification [9].

It is crucial that models exposed to health data follow strict de-identification, secure training, and data governance. Health data is very private, especially those associated with patients. Fortunately, regulatory expectations are evolving as agencies like the FDA are publishing lifecycle guidance for AI/ML in medical devices [13], however, approval pathways and post-market monitoring practices are still maturing. Providers must document intended use and human oversight. Organizations planning clinical deployment must evaluate whether an LLM-based function qualifies as a medical device under the respective regulations and follow submission/lifecycle recommendations [13]. Meanwhile the European Union focuses on the EU AI Act [12], which imposes strict regulations on medical applications.

Finally, the LLMs must be integrated into the clinical workflow and have to build trust. Poor UX, misaligned outputs, or trivialization of clinician expertise can reduce adoption or cause harm. Checking the implementation and its adoption regularly is essential and can, e.g., be achieved by monitoring the usage via log files [29].

16.1.7 Practices for Safe Implementation

Most importantly, the intended use and risk class, i.e., clinical aid vs. autonomous decision, need to be defined. [12, 13]. Instead of "pure" LLMs, RAG should be preferred. Models can be connected to verified internal knowledge bases and show sources to reduce hallucinations [2]. Details will be discussed in a later section.

A human-in-the-loop approach should be considered as a further safety measure. It requires that clinicians review for any output that affects diagnosis/treatment [18]. Additionally, local validation and monitoring is a very good option. This can be used for prospective evaluation in the population, continuous performance monitoring, and feedback loops [29].

Finally, it is a good idea to make use of encryption, de-identification, and contractual protections for models trained on patient data [12, 13] to avoid any possible problems with data governance and privacy. Logging the used prompt, their respective output, and clinician actions contributes significantly to safety and liability [9].

16.1.8 New Opportunities for LLM in Healthcare

Apart from all challenges, there are massive opportunities in leveraging LLM technology in healthcare. Some ideas have been created but have not yet been completely implemented and verified.

The question whether LLM-enabled interventions improve patient morbidity, mortality, or health equity still needs to be proven on a clinical level. So far, large multisite RCTs are limited [9]. There has been some research on fine-tuning on local data and dealing with distribution shift [46]. However, the robustness and domain adaptation of this approach need to be proven, leading to optimized methods for continuous updating.

From a UX perspective, human factors need to be considered. A good method would be to observe how clinicians interact with LLMs under time pressure and cognitive load [29]. Finally, regulatory evaluation metrics may not be neglected. Standardized benchmarks that reflect safety-critical clinical tasks rather than only exam-style QA are the topic of current research [47].

16.2 Speech-Based Documentation with LLMs

16.2.1 Introduction

Speech-based documentation systems—often called ambient AI scribes or AI-powered clinical documentation assistants [30]—pair automated speech recognition (ASR) with natural-language understanding and LLMs to transcribe and convert clinician–patient conversations into clinical notes.

Recent multi-site pilots and the first randomized clinical trial(s) of LLM-powered ambient scribes report modest but meaningful reductions in documentation time, improvements in clinician workflow and satisfaction in some settings [33], and a rapidly expanding commercial adoption [32, 48]. However, important caveats remain: sometimes modest accuracy (speech recognition and LLM summarization), hallucination/factual errors, privacy/PHI risk, and limited evidence linking deployment to improved patient outcomes [27]. Key recent studies showing these points include the first randomized clinical trial of two ambient AI scribes, several multi-site implementation reports (including large health systems), and systematic reviews of AI-based speech/documentation tools [37].

16.2.2 Components and Workflows

There is a variety of technologies included, from the audio ingestion of clinical encounters (live or recorded), the actual ASR, and the use of LLMs/NLP to summarize, structure, and output clinical documentation (notes, problem lists, orders, patient instructions). Typically, these are arranged in a pipeline (see Fig. 16.1). Capabilities, evidence, implementation patterns, risks, regulatory considerations, evaluation metrics, and recommendations must be addressed and are discussed in the following sections.

16.2.3 Capabilities of Current Systems

This section illustrates for which tasks speech-based systems can be used and their specific advantages. The most crucial capability is the tremendous speed increase for basic documentation. Spoken encounters can be converted to draft notes very efficiently and quickly, which reduces repetitive typing and allows focusing on the really difficult problems. Also, automatically filled structured fields (e.g., medications, vitals) and generated discharge instructions prove to be a valuable optimization provided by LLMs.

But it is not only internal templates and reports that can be filled in automatically; vendors increasingly provide specialty-specific templates and include models to improve phrasing and relevance. This must be integrated into the clinical workflow. Some solutions already integrate directly with major EHRs (API or vendor partnerships). These capabilities are well documented in large-scale deployments and product evaluations [32, 34].

16.2.4 Examples of Current Use

Some of the first pragmatic randomized trials comparing two ambient AI scribes (Microsoft DAX and Nabla) to usual care found modest reductions in time-in-note and mixed effects on clinician burnout metrics; the trials also highlight usability and error-detection needs. The first RCT evidence for LLM-powered ambient scribe tools is a milestone achievement [32].

Large health systems, e.g. [42], report rapid adoption with millions of uses and substantial time savings and clinician satisfaction in some specialties but emphasize careful rollout, consent processes, and monitoring. On the implementation side, reports show big operational gains but at the same time note the need for governance [7, 48].

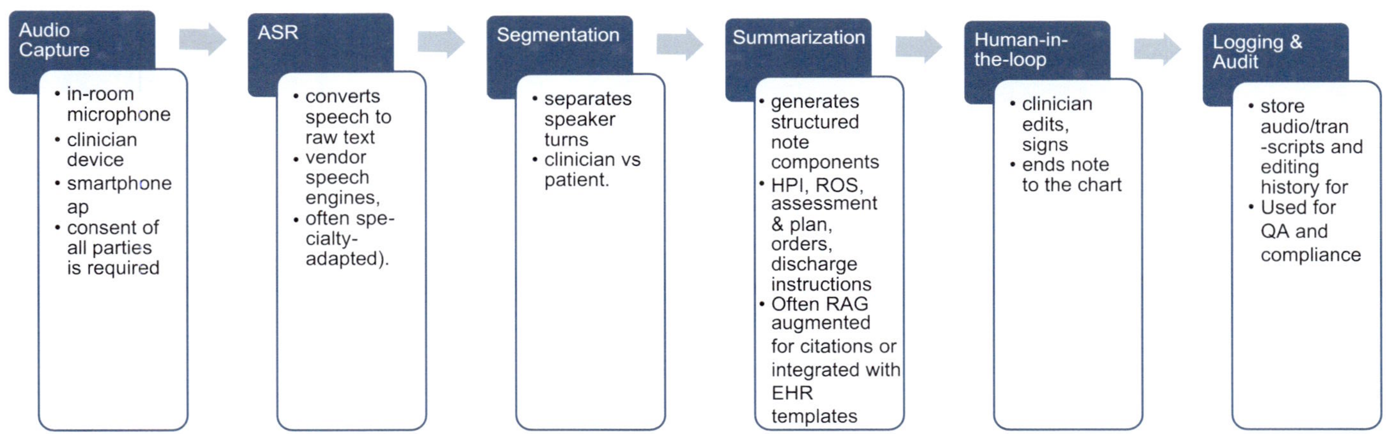

Fig. 16.1 Typical pipeline

Several single-site evaluations of products like Nuance DAX, Dragon Medical, and other commercial tools show mixed results—some efficiency gains, others showing no statistically significant improvement for certain productivity measures. Accuracy and clinical quality vary by specialty, encounter type, and local workflow integration [20, 55].

Recent systematic reviews and evaluation frameworks examine ASR and LLM systems' technical performance, human factors, and ethical/regulatory gaps. They stress that standardized evaluation metrics like time, edits, accuracy, safety events, and equity need to be evaluated carefully [37, 53].

16.2.5 Key Advantages and Expected Benefits

The technology can support existing processes and make them more effective and efficient. Multiple reports and deployments document reduced clinician documentation time, which leads to improved work–life balance in many cases. Moreover, work happiness grows as routine tasks take less time [7, 48]. This also has implications for patients, as clinicians report being able to focus more on patients' needs when not having to spend too much time on documentation. Qualitative interviews show a positive perceived impact on patient engagement [45]. Finally, ambient AI scribes promise greater scalability and cheaper per-visit cost compared to hiring specialized human scribes [35]. The saved costs can be invested otherwise.

16.2.6 Risks and Potential Failures

Although the technology is already quite sophisticated and has proved valuable in other domains, there are some risks involved in the implementation. Mis-transcribed words (medical terms, names, numbers) can introduce dangerous inaccuracies if not corrected during automatic speech recognition. Accuracy depends on audio quality, accents, specialty vocabulary, and background noise, but also on the quality of the software and models used. Models may perform worse with non-standard accents, non-English languages, or underrepresented subpopulations, risking inequitable documentation quality. Moreover, during speech recognition, a statement might be misattributed (clinician/patient ambiguity) and can create inaccurate history or orders [37]).

A structural problem arises when LLMs invent facts (e.g., assert exam findings not said, infer wrong duration or dosing). Without reliable grounding and clinician review, these hallucination errors can be propagated. Several implementation studies and reviews flag this as a core safety concern [37].

Audio and intermediate transcripts are PHI; storing and transmitting them to cloud vendors introduces both legal and contractual risks. Therefore, consent, encryption, and data governance are essential [43]. Also, (local) regulations need to be considered. Whether an ambient scribe or an LLM-generated note constitutes a medical device or clinical decision support varies by jurisdiction and by the product's intended claims; liability for errors (clinician vs vendor) is not fully settled. Regulatory frameworks and guidance are rapidly evolving [5, 53].

16.2.7 Implementation and Deployment

Typically, a project is arranged in distinctive phases as can be seen in Fig. 16.2.

Before the actual implementation, a project governance must be established by creating, e.g., a multidisciplinary steering group (clinicians, IT, privacy, legal, QI, patient reps). The use cases need to be defined, and it's often best to start with low-risk specialties/visit types (e.g., primary care follow-ups, non-procedural visits) and specific documentation tasks (note drafting, problem list suggestions). If (software) vendors are involved, due diligence checks need to be performed. Typical (vendor) documents supporting that can be model cards, training-data provenance, ASR word-error rates on clinical speech, privacy controls, and SOC/HIPAA compliance. If patients are involved, getting their consent is crucial, e.g., for audio capture where required by law or institution policy [48].

The deployment itself needs to start with a *verification* of all AI-generated notes by clinicians, which is directly followed by a (pilot) acceptance test. Canonical test cases should be conceived for verifying ASR accuracy and specialty-specific prompts, hallucination challenge sets, and equity testing (accent/language subsets). Logging and auditing are crucial and can be achieved by storing both the original audio and ASR transcript, LLM drafts and the edit history, and final note for QA and regulatory purposes. Finally, data security must be considered. Typical measures include data encryption, limited retention policies, and role-based access controls [48].

Finally, after the solution is in production, it needs to be carefully monitored and maintained. For this, a real-time monitoring dashboard can be used to look at time-saved metrics, edits/note, hallucination incident rate, and clinician feedback. This feedback should be integrated into the feedback loop to enable clinicians to flag errors and propagate this to vendor/model updates. As models and software tend to change, a periodic revalidation after software updates or model changes is

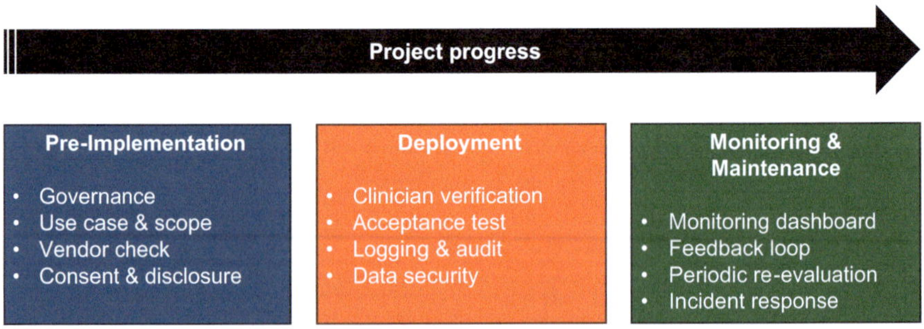

Fig. 16.2 Project phases

necessary, both pre- and post-release. If incidents occur, a predefined process for investigating and remediating must start as soon as possible and include the AI output [53].

16.2.8 Ethical, Legal & Regulatory Notes

As conversations between clinicians and patients are analyzed, ethical and legal considerations must be taken into account. Audio capture often contains sensitive, privacy-relevant data. Therefore, it must follow local laws (e.g., one-party vs. two-party consent) and institutional policies. Explicit patient opt-out workflows are recommended [43]. Some deployments (if they make diagnostic or therapeutic claims) may be considered medical devices where local regulations might apply [13]. Therefore, it is crucial to engage regulatory/compliance teams early. Evaluation and post-market surveillance expectations are increasing [53]. AI often has a reputation of being untransparent. To overcome this, clear UI signals that the document was created with AI assistance must be included.

16.3 Conversational AI and Medical Chatbots

16.3.1 Introduction

Conversational AI (chatbots, virtual assistants, and voice agents) is rapidly becoming a mainstream tool in healthcare for patient triage, mental-health support, administrative automation, medication adherence, and clinician-assist functions. Randomized and controlled studies—especially in mental health and history-taking—show promising clinical and operational benefits, e.g., reduced symptom scores, faster intake, but evidence on improved hard clinical outcomes like morbidity and mortality is limited and heterogeneous. Major risks remain: safety (halluci nations, incorrect triage) [33], privacy (PHI in chat logs), equity (worse performance for underrepresented languages/accents), and regulatory uncertainty. Regulatory bodies like the FDA have published lifecycle guidance for AI-enabled device software functions [13], increasing expectations for transparency, monitoring, and post-market surveillance. Health systems should treat conversational AI as high-value but high-risk—pilot narrowly, require human-in-the-loop oversight for clinical tasks, and use rigorous evaluation and monitoring before scaling [27, 30, 47].

16.3.2 Architectures & Flavors

Conversational AI systems vary along three axes as can be seen in Fig. 16.3.

The task intent can be, e.g., patient-facing triage or symptom checkers with automated routing. This is realized by therapeutic chatbots like Woebot [57], Wysa [58], and Youper [60]. On the other hand, administrative voice agents can make insurance

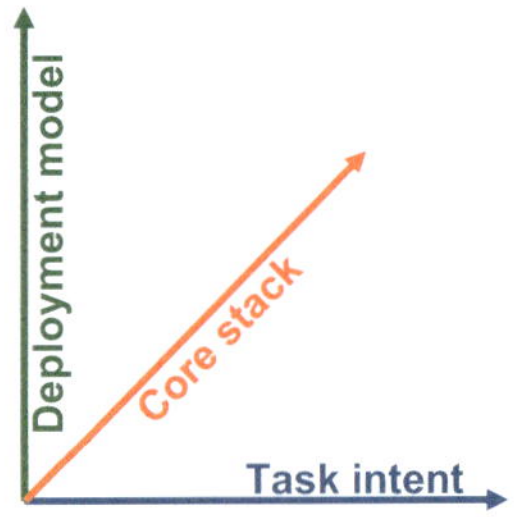

Fig. 16.3 Conversation AI dimensions

calls or schedule appointments. Moreover, the systems can support clinicians by note drafting or question answering.

In the core stack, ASR is used for converting voice recordings to text. Responses can be created by generative LLMs supported by rules. RAG (see later section) grounds outputs in knowledge bases.

This technology can be deployed in closed, domain-adapted models with local data or vendor-hosted LLMs. Hybrid designs facilitate the combination of scripted triage with generative fallback. A pure cloud scenario where everything is running in the cloud is also possible.

16.3.3 Historic and Current Usage (Table 16.2)

Today, there is a focus on various solutions and domains:

Scalable CBT and supportive conversations are used in mental health and chat therapy; several RCTs/meta-analyses show small-to-moderate reductions in anxiety/depression symptoms [30, 62]. Self-triage apps guide users to the appropriate level of care and check symptoms; mixed accuracy vs clinicians and varied conservative/over-triage tendencies can be observed [33].

Chatbots collect structured histories and social-determinant screenings in clinical intake and patient history; this improves completeness and standardization [24]. Automated insurance calls help relieve administrative burden; voice agents support prior-authorization tasks. Scheduling, and benefits verification show operational ROI in some case studies [54]. Medication reminders are used for patient navigation, chronic care engagement, symptom monitoring, and resource navigation bots [4].

16.3.4 Literature Review

Some solutions are already in operation, with researchers reporting different success rates. Multiple RCTs and meta-analyses demonstrate reductions in anxiety and depressive symptoms vs. control conditions, though effect sizes and durability vary [27, 62]. Additionally, conversational AI can improve completeness and efficiency of medical history-taking. Systematic reviews report improved data collection and

Table 16.2 Development of LLM-based chatbots in healthcare over time

2010–2015	Rule-based chatbots and symptom checkers
2016–2020	ML/NLU-based virtual assistants in administrative workflows
2020–2023	Scalable mental-health chatbots (Woebot, Wysa) collect RCT evidence for short-term symptom reduction [27]
2023–2025	LLMs and multimodal models expand conversational capabilities; studies compare LLM triage/QA to clinicians and examine hallucination/triage performance. Regulatory agencies publish lifecycle guidance for AI-enabled medical devices [12, 21]

patient satisfaction in certain settings [24]. However, triage accuracy of LLMs and chatbots is mixed. Large models can triage reasonably but often differ from clinician judgment; some studies find LLMs over- or under-triage compared to professionals. This heterogeneity demands local validation before clinical use [33].

Deployment evidence is dominated by single-site pilots; only a few multisite pragmatic RCTs measure hard clinical outcomes. Reviews call for larger, rigorously designed pragmatic trials with patient-centered endpoints [25, 30]. At the same time, regulators are tightening expectations. The FDA and other agencies now expect total-product-lifecycle management, transparency, bias testing, and post-market surveillance for AI-enabled medical devices [21].

16.3.5 Benefits, Limitations, & Risks

The new technology has a lot of benefits. The systems are very scalable and offer both 24/7 access and lower marginal cost per interaction [26]. By improving access and using equity potential, they can reach underserved areas or times when clinicians aren't available [52]. Standardization makes sure that intake remains consistent, while checklist completion ensures the reliability of screening tasks [24].

However, there are some important limitations and risks. Generative models can produce plausible but incorrect medical statements. RAG and conservative policies help but do not completely eliminate the risk [1, 33], as will be shown in the next section. Chat logs and audio are PHI and therefore sensitive information; the storage and vendor data usage must meet HIPAA and local laws [12, 13]. ASR and NLU often perform worse for non-native accents, underrepresented languages, and certain demographic groups, which makes equity audits essential [3]. Finally, regulatory and legal requirements need to be met. Classification as clinical decision support or medical device depends on claims and uses; liability boundaries are still unclear [14, 56].

The FDA (and other regulators) issued draft and final guidance emphasizing lifecycle oversight for AI/ML-enabled medical software, transparency, and bias mitigation; developers may be required to submit more detailed documentation depending on claims and risk. Jurisdictions differ in definitions and thresholds. Engage regulatory/compliance teams early [12, 21].

16.3.6 Implementation

The following steps are recommended for an implementation:

1. *Define intended use and perform risk classification*:
   differentiate between informational, diagnostic, and therapeutic use cases [13].
2. *Require provenance and grounding*:
   for medical claims, use RAG and cite sources where possible [1].
3. *Human-in-the-loop for clinical decisions*:
   mandate clinician review for high-risk outputs.
4. *Data governance and consent*:
   ensure explicit consent, retention limits, encryption, vendor contracts with HIPAA/SOC2 [13].
5. *Equity and robustness testing*:
   test across languages, accents, and subpopulations [3].
6. *Monitoring and incident response*:
   implement real-time dashboards, error flagging, and rapid rollback plans [14].

16.4 Enhancing Trustworthiness with RAG

16.4.1 Introduction

RAG—the pattern of retrieving authoritative, domain-specific content and supplying it as context to a generative LLM—is one of the most promising practical strategies to improve LLM trustworthiness in healthcare. RAG improves factuality, enables provenance (source linking), reduces hallucinations on many tasks, and lets organizations constrain models to current, local, and regulated knowledge (guidelines, formularies, and charts). Recent empirical work across radiology, medication safety, surgical guidance, and broader LLM evaluations shows substantial gains in accuracy and reduction of dangerous errors when RAG is used and properly engineered. However, RAG is not a silver bullet: retrieval quality, index freshness, prompt & answer verification, privacy of retrieval sources, and system-level workflows remain critical [2, 59].

RAG combines two main components: The retriever is a fast module (vector retrieval with sparse or dense vectors) that searches a knowledge corpus (guidelines, local EHR notes, drug formularies, literature, and all kinds of documents) and returns a small set of relevant documents or passages. The generator is a large generative language model. It consumes the retrieved context plus the user query (prompt) to produce an answer. Optionally, the generator is instructed to quote or cite retrieved passages and to be conservative when no high-confidence retrieval exists.

There are some popular variants of RAG. In closed-index RAG, the index is built from local, controlled sources (hospital guidelines, drug database). This is the best option for safety and PHI control. Hybrid RAG combines the local index with public knowledge sources (like websites) for up-to-date coverage and is also able to answer generic questions. To avoid hallucinations, a RAG pipeline can include a reranker for narrowing the list of potential results and an additional verification stage that detects exactly those hallucinations [2, 31].

RAG helps by providing explicit, up-to-date evidence to the LLM at generation time and constrains the output while enabling provenance linking (citations). All this helps to reduce the model's tendency to invent facts and makes outputs auditable [61]. Moreover, updating content in RAG systems is much easier compared to fine-tuning a generative LLM.

16.4.2 Mechanisms for Improving Trustworthiness

RAG has several mechanisms that increase trustworthiness. The most important point is the reduction of hallucinations. Empirical studies show markedly fewer fabricated facts when responses are grounded on retrieved texts rather than pure prior models. For example, RAG significantly reduced hallucinations in radiology contrast guidance and other clinical vignettes [22, 51]. The reason is that the generative LLM is not used as a knowledge base but rather as a summarizer. Moreover, RAG enables provenance and transparency. Retrieved passages can be shown as citations or links, enabling clinicians to verify claims and auditors to trace recommendations to sources [2].

On the operational side, RAG makes sure that knowledge is kept current, as it can query up-to-date documents (EHR notes, recent guidelines), bypassing model training cutoffs or fine-tuning. Studies benchmarking LLM workflows with RAG report better performance on time-sensitive tasks [15]. This facilitates domain adaptation; indexing local protocols or formulary content makes outputs reflect institutional practice, increasing relevance and reducing harmful mismatch. Case studies (e.g., MedLM/RAG integrations) report operational improvements when local knowledge is used [17]. In addition to that, the database can stay on-premise.

Empirical results look great. A recent study reported RAG-enhanced local models eliminated dangerous hallucinations for radiology contrast questions and outperformed cloud LLM baselines on safety metrics [22]. This is achieved by taking a look at only trusted sources. Multi-model assessments show RAG variants outperform plain LLMs for tasks like preoperative instruction generation and surgical-fitness assessment across multiple guidelines [28]. The much narrower database contributes to the improved results. ClinicalRAG and other academic pipelines demonstrate improved reference ability and decision-support performance in experimental benchmarks [31]. This helps in constructing an audit trail.

16.4.3 RAG Architecture and Engineering Patterns

There is no reference architecture, but some practical aspects are considered by [2, 44] and depicted in Fig. 16.4:

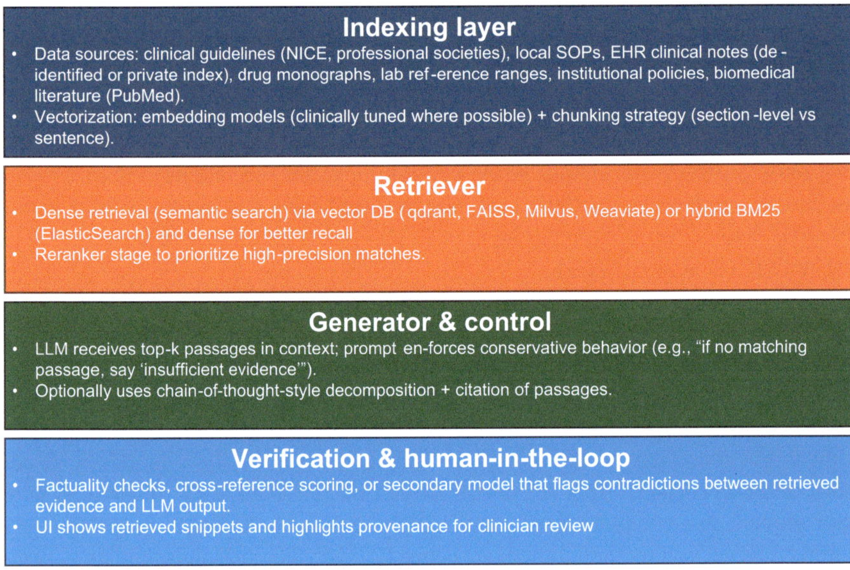

Fig. 16.4 RAG architecture in healthcare

It turns out that engineering is critical [2]. Retrieval length should be limited, and a chunking strategy should be chosen that preserves clinical context (e.g., entire guideline section vs. sentence). Where it is possible, domain-specific embedding models (biomedical embeddings) should be used, and recall on clinical queries must be calculated as a KPI. To further improve trustworthiness, a fallback policy (decline to answer or defer) should be in place when retrieval confidence is low.

16.4.4 Risks and Potential Failures

RAG reduces but does not eliminate risks. Possible failures can still occur; the most important with possible cures are listed with the most frequent at the top below:

1. *Retrieval errors (garbage in—garbage out)*

   If the retriever returns irrelevant or outdated passages, the generative model will still produce wrong answers. This can be avoided first of all by a high quality of the underlying text corpus (maybe with the help of data curation). A reranker can act as a safeguard and calculate retrieval confidence thresholds; frequent index refreshes should be applied to update outdated information [2].
2. *Citation misuse/selective quoting*

   The generative model might still paraphrase inaccurately or selectively combine passages to create misleading synthesis. Possible cures include requiring verbatim quotes for critical facts, showing the exact retrieved snippets, and implementing conservative answer policies. It is crucial to measure failure rates to permanently avoid this issue.

3. *Index privacy and PHI leakage*
   Indexing raw EHR text can expose PHI to vector databases or cloud vendors (if not hosting on-premise). This is especially critical if not only the vectors but also the corresponding texts are saved in the database. This situation can be avoided by keeping clinical indices on-premise, by encrypting the index storage (also possible in the cloud), by applying de-identification where appropriate, or by imposing contractual controls [2].
4. *Outdated or conflicting sources*
   Multiple guidelines may disagree on which RAG to retrieve, and the model may not resolve conflicts correctly. A possible cure might be to tag sources by authority and date and present possible conflicts actively to the users. A model that transparently tells users conflicting text passages with references increases its trustworthiness tremendously ([28], p. 10).
5. *Over-reliance on retrieval confidence*
   Retrieval confidence metrics can be imperfect, which means that systems still require human oversight for high-risk outputs. This cannot be totally avoided, but the problem can be shown as uncertainty to users via a conservative UI/UX. The system then still needs a human-in-the-loop signoff for diagnosis/treatment [2].
6. *Device classification and claims*
   If the RAG system makes diagnostic/treatment recommendations or automates clinical decisions, regulators (e.g., FDA) may classify it as a medical device (SaMD). Claims must be supported by clinical evidence and lifecycle plans. Therefore, it is useful to focus on regulatory and legal teams early [12, 13, 38].
7. *Transparency and documentation*
   Models and their performance can change. Therefore, maintaining model cards and keeping data provenance records is crucial. Moreover, a copy of the retrieval index should be kept, as well as release notes describing index refresh policy. These aid audits and post-market surveillance [59].

16.4.5 Evaluation and Acceptance Tests

To validate an RAG system before clinical use, a structured evaluation should be adopted.

In the offline technical validation, a few KPIs can be measured or calculated. The retrieval recall should be calculated for a gold set of clinical questions to measure whether the retriever returns relevant passages in top-k (recall@k). The citation accuracy measures the fraction of model statements that are supported verbatim by a retrieved passage (precision of citations). With the help of the hallucination rate, the number of fabricated or unverifiable claims per 1000 responses on a curated clinical test set can be measured [8].

In the clinical simulation phase, case vignettes should be used to present simulated or de-identified cases and measure clinical correctness (diagnosis, med dosing, contraindication detection) compared to expert panel. Studies show that RAG improves the detection of medication errors vs. using a generative model alone [39].

User acceptance and safety are critical during operation. This can be measured via the clinician editing burden (e.g., via edits per draft, time-to-sign). The provable provenance is the percentage of outputs with explicit, clickable citations to institutional policies. As an escalation and fallback measure, the correct triggering of escalation for low-confidence cases should be recorded.

Further metrics should be considered while the solution is in use. Real-world incidents where RAG output contributed to clinical action should be tracked. The system should be prepared for rapid review and rollback ahead of each deployment [15].

Of course, the metrics vary by use case and institution. Some example criteria could look like this: Retrieval recall@5 ≥90% on a curated guideline retrieval test. Citation precision ≥95% for medication and dosing statements. Hallucination rate <1 per 1000 high-risk outputs in simulated tests. Clinician net satisfaction ≥ baseline and no severe safety incidents in initial 60-day pilot.

16.4.6 Case Studies

RAG adoption is progressing very fast. Some examples have already been published.

A local RAG approach eliminated hallucinations in 100 synthetic radiology cases and outperformed cloud LLMs on safety metrics. The study highlights how on-premise RAG with local indexes protects PHI while improving safety [22, 51]. Multimodal RAG is also gaining traction. Such an assessment across many guidelines showed RAG workflows produced more consistent and guideline-concordant outputs than LLMs alone [28]. Safety is always an issue in health, and RAG adoption can contribute to increasing this, especially when less experienced people are involved. RAG-LLM pipelines used alongside junior pharmacists improved detection of drug-related problems versus LLM alone in vignettes spanning 12 specialties [39]. Open-source plays an important role both with respect to models and implementations. Using this approach, prototypes can demonstrate how to extract heterogeneous clinical knowledge and combine it into RAG workflows for CDS [31].

These case studies collectively show consistent direction: anchoring generative LLMs to trustworthy sources raises factuality and clinical usefulness, particularly for well-scoped tasks.

References

1. Abbasian M, Khatibi E, Azimi I, Oniani D, Shakeri Hossein Abad Z, Thieme A, Sriram R, Yang Z, Wang Y, Lin B, Gevaert O, Li L-J, Jain R, Rahmani AM. Foundation metrics for evaluating effectiveness of healthcare conversations powered by generative AI. NPJ Digit Med. 2024;7(1):82. https://doi.org/10.1038/s41746-024-01074-z.
2. Amugongo LM, Mascheroni P, Brooks S, Doering S, Seidel J. Retrieval augmented generation for large language models in healthcare: a systematic review. PLOS Digit Health. 2025;4(6):e0000877. https://doi.org/10.1371/journal.pdig.0000877.

3. Augenstein J, Seigel R, Shashoua M, Irlbeck C. Manatt Health: Health AI policy tracker. 2025. https://www.manatt.com/insights/newsletters/health-highlights/manatt-health-health-ai-policy-tracker
4. Authors, Clark M, Bailey S. Chatbots in health care: connecting patients to information: emerging health technologies. Canadian Agency for Drugs and Technologies in Health; 2024. http://www.ncbi.nlm.nih.gov/books/NBK602381/.
5. Balloch J, Sridharan S, Oldham G, Wray J, Gough P, Robinson R, Sebire NJ, Khalil S, Asgari E, Tan C, Taylor A, Pimenta D. Use of an ambient artificial intelligence tool to improve quality of clinical documentation. Future Healthc J. 2024;11(3):100157. https://doi.org/10.1016/j.fhj.2024.100157.
6. Brown TB, Mann B, Ryder N, Subbiah M, Kaplan J, Dhariwal P, Neelakantan A, Shyam P, Sastry G, Askell A, Agarwal S, Herbert-Voss A, Krueger G, Henighan T, Child R, Ramesh A, Ziegler DM, Wu J, Winter C, et al. Language models are few-shot learners (no. arXiv:2005.14165). arXiv. 2020; https://doi.org/10.48550/arXiv.2005.14165.
7. Bruce G. 16K hours saved: ambient AI scribes at Kaiser Permanente. Becker's Hospital Review | Healthcare News & Analysis. 2025. https://www.beckershospitalreview.com/healthcare-information-technology/ai/16k-hours-saved-ambient-ai-scribes-at-kaiser-permanente/.
8. Bunnell DJ, Bondy MJ, Fromtling LM, Ludeman E, Gourab K. Bridging AI and healthcare: a scoping review of retrieval-augmented generation—ethics, bias, transparency, improvements, and applications. medRxiv. 2025:2025.04.01.25325033. https://doi.org/10.1101/2025.04.01.25325033.
9. Busch F, Hoffmann L, Rueger C, van Dijk EH, Kader R, Ortiz-Prado E, Makowski MR, Saba L, Hadamitzky M, Kather JN, Truhn D, Cuocolo R, Adams LC, Bressem KK. Current applications and challenges in large language models for patient care: a systematic review. Commun Med. 2025;5(1):26. https://doi.org/10.1038/s43856-024-00717-2.
10. Corrado G, Barral J. Advancing medical AI with Med-Gemini. 2024. https://research.google/blog/advancing-medical-ai-with-med-gemini/.
11. Eriksen AV, Möller S, Ryg J. Use of GPT-4 to diagnose complex clinical cases. NEJM AI. 2024;1(1):AIp2300031. https://doi.org/10.1056/AIp2300031.
12. EU AI Act: First regulation on artificial intelligence. Topics | European Parliament. 2023. https://www.europarl.europa.eu/topics/en/article/20230601STO93804/eu-ai-act-first-regulation-on-artificial-intelligence.
13. FDA. Artificial intelligence in software as a medical device. FDA. 2025. https://www.fda.gov/medical-devices/software-medical-device-samd/artificial-intelligence-software-medical-device.
14. Freyer O, Wiest IC, Kather JN, Gilbert S. A future role for health applications of large language models depends on regulators enforcing safety standards. Lancet Digit Health. 2024;6(9):e662–72. https://doi.org/10.1016/S2589-7500(24)00124-9.
15. Gaber F, Shaik M, Allega F, Bilecz AJ, Busch F, Goon K, Franke V, Akalin A. Evaluating large language model workflows in clinical decision support for triage and referral and diagnosis. Npj Digit Med. 2025;8(1):263. https://doi.org/10.1038/s41746-025-01684-1.
16. Garcia P, Ma SP, Shah S, Smith M, Jeong Y, Devon-Sand A, Tai-Seale M, Takazawa K, Clutter D, Vogt K, Lugtu C, Rojo M, Lin S, Shanafelt T, Pfeffer MA, Sharp C. Artificial Intelligence–generated draft replies to patient inbox messages. JAMA Netw Open. 2024;7(3):e243201. https://doi.org/10.1001/jamanetworkopen.2024.3201.
17. GM A, Dhar G. Apollo 24|7 uses MedLM and RAG for healthcare innovation. Google Cloud Blog. n.d. Retrieved August 13, 2025, from https://cloud.google.com/blog/products/ai-machine-learning/how-apollo-247-leverages-medlm-with-rag-to-revolutionize-healthcare.
18. Goh E, Gallo R, Hom J, Strong E, Weng Y, Kerman H, Cool JA, Kanjee Z, Parsons AS, Ahuja N, Horvitz E, Yang D, Milstein A, Olson APJ, Rodman A, Chen JH. Large language model influence on diagnostic reasoning: a randomized clinical trial. JAMA Netw Open. 2024;7(10):e2440969. https://doi.org/10.1001/jamanetworkopen.2024.40969.
19. Google. Med-PaLM: a medical large language model - Google Research. 2022. https://sites.research.google/med-palm/.

20. Haberle T, Cleveland C, Snow GL, Barber C, Stookey N, Thornock C, Younger L, Mullahkhel B, Ize-Ludlow D. The impact of nuance DAX ambient listening AI documentation: a cohort study. J Am Med Inform Assoc. 2024;31(4):975–9. https://doi.org/10.1093/jamia/ocae022.
21. Health, C. for D. and R. Artificial intelligence in software as a medical device. FDA. 2025. https://www.fda.gov/medical-devices/software-medical-device-samd/artificial-intelligence-software-medical-device.
22. Healthcare in Europe. Eliminating LLM hallucinations in radiology with RAG. 2025. https://healthcare-in-europe.com/en/news/eliminate-llm-hallucinations-radiology-rag.html.
23. Hersh W. Artificial intelligence: implications for healthcare practice, research, and education. 2025.
24. Hindelang M, Sitaru S, Zink A. Transforming Health care through Chatbots for medical history-taking and future directions: comprehensive systematic review. JMIR Med Inform. 2024;12(1):e56628. https://doi.org/10.2196/56628.
25. Jacob C, Brasier N, Laurenzi E, Heuss S, Mougiakakou S-G, Cöltekin A, Peter MK. AI for IMPACTS framework for evaluating the long-term real-world impacts of AI-powered clinician tools: systematic review and narrative synthesis. J Med Internet Res. 2025;27(1):e67485. https://doi.org/10.2196/67485.
26. Jeon H. Can an AI Chatbot become your therapist? We had real people put it to the test. Prevention; 2025. https://www.prevention.com/health/mental-health/a65045817/mental-health-ai-chatbots-therapy/.
27. Karkosz S, Szymański R, Sanna K, Michałowski J. Effectiveness of a web-based and mobile therapy Chatbot on anxiety and depressive symptoms in subclinical young adults: randomized controlled trial. JMIR Formative Res. 2024;8:e47960. https://doi.org/10.2196/47960.
28. Ke YH, Jin L, Elangovan K, Abdullah HR, Liu N, Sia ATH, Soh CR, Tung JYM, Ong JCL, Kuo C-F, Wu S-C, Kovacheva VP, Ting DSW. Retrieval augmented generation for 10 large language models and its generalizability in assessing medical fitness. Npj Digit Med. 2025;8(1):187. https://doi.org/10.1038/s41746-025-01519-z.
29. Li H, Fu J-F, Python A. Implementing large language models in health care: clinician-focused review with interactive guideline. J Med Internet Res. 2025;27(1):e71916. https://doi.org/10.2196/71916.
30. Li H, Zhang R, Lee Y-C, Kraut RE, Mohr DC. Systematic review and meta-analysis of AI-based conversational agents for promoting mental health and well-being. Npj Digit Med. 2023;6(1):236. https://doi.org/10.1038/s41746-023-00979-5.
31. Lu Y, Zhao X, Wang J. ClinicalRAG: enhancing clinical decision support through heterogeneous knowledge retrieval. In: Li S, Li M, Zhang MJ, Choi E, Geva M, Hase P, Ji H, editors. Proceedings of the 1st workshop on towards knowledgeable language models (KnowLLM 2024). Association for Computational Linguistics; 2024. p. 64–8. https://doi.org/10.18653/v1/2024.knowllm-1.6.
32. Lukac PJ, Turner W, Vangala S, Chin AT, Khalili J, Shih Y-CT, Sarkisian C, Cheng EM, Mafi JN. A randomized-clinical trial of two ambient artificial intelligence scribes: measuring documentation efficiency and physician burnout. medRxiv: The Preprint Server for Health Sciences. 2025:2025.07.10.25331333. https://doi.org/10.1101/2025.07.10.25331333.
33. Masanneck L, Schmidt L, Seifert A, Kölsche T, Huntemann N, Jansen R, Mehsin M, Bernhard M, Meuth SG, Böhm L, Pawlitzki M. Triage performance across large language models, ChatGPT, and untrained doctors in emergency Medicine: comparative study. J Med Internet Res. 2024;26(1):e53297. https://doi.org/10.2196/53297.
34. Microsoft. Dragon Medical One | Microsoft Cloud for Healthcare. n.d. Retrieved August 13, 2025, from https://www.microsoft.com/en-us/health-solutions/clinical-workflow/dragon-medical-one.
35. Murgia M. Healthcare turns to AI for medical note-taking 'scribes'. Financial Times. 2025; https://www.ft.com/content/5c356658-6db4-47c1-940b-b2e3cf3a51f3.
36. Narang S, Chowdhery A. Pathways Language Model (PaLM): scaling to 540 billion parameters for breakthrough. 2022. https://research.google/blog/pathways-language-model-palm-scaling-to-540-billion-parameters-for-breakthrough-performance/.

37. Ng JJW, Wang E, Zhou X, Zhou KX, Goh CXL, Sim GZN, Tan HK, Goh SSN, Ng QX. Evaluating the performance of artificial intelligence-based speech recognition for clinical documentation: a systematic review. BMC Med Inform Decis Mak. 2025a;25:236. https://doi.org/10.1186/s12911-025-03061-0.
38. Ng KKY, Matsuba I, Zhang PC. RAG in health care: a novel framework for improving communication and decision-making by addressing LLM limitations. NEJM AI. 2025b;2(1):AIra2400380. https://doi.org/10.1056/AIra2400380.
39. Ong JCL, Jin L, Elangovan K, Lim GYS, Lim DYZ, Sng GGR, Ke Y, Tung JYM, Zhong RJ, Koh CMY, Lee KZH, Chen X, Chng JK, Than A, Goh KJ, Ting DSW. Development and testing of a novel large language model-based clinical decision support systems for medication safety in 12 clinical specialties (no. arXiv:2402.01741). arXiv. 2024; https://doi.org/10.48550/arXiv.2402.01741.
40. Open AI. Introducing ChatGPT. 2022. https://openai.com/index/chatgpt/.
41. Parthasarathy VB, Zafar A, Khan A, Shahid A. The ultimate guide to fine-tuning LLMs from basics to breakthroughs: an exhaustive review of technologies, research, best practices, applied research challenges and opportunities (No. arXiv:2408.13296; Version 1). arXiv. 2024; https://doi.org/10.48550/arXiv.2408.13296.
42. Permanente Medicine. Permanente medical groups. Permanente Medicine. n.d. Retrieved August 14, 2025, from https://permanente.org/permanente-medical-groups/.
43. Peterson Health Technology Institute. Adoption of artificial intelligence in healthcare delivery systems: early applications and impacts. Peterson Health Technology Institute; 2025. https://phti.org/ai-adoption-early-applications-impacts/.
44. Pinna S, Massa SM, Fenu M, Casti G, Riboni D. Integration of retrieval-augmented generation technique for LLM-based differential diagnosis assistant. In: Proceedings of the 18th ACM international conference on PErvasive technologies related to assistive environments; 2025. p. 277–84. https://doi.org/10.1145/3733155.3733192.
45. Shah SJ, Crowell T, Jeong Y, Devon-Sand A, Smith M, Yang B, Ma SP, Liang AS, Delahaie C, Hsia C, Shanafelt T, Pfeffer MA, Sharp C, Lin S, Garcia P. Physician perspectives on ambient AI scribes. JAMA Netw Open. 2025;8(3):e251904. https://doi.org/10.1001/jamanetworkopen.2025.1904.
46. Singh V, Cheng S, Kwan AC, Ebinger J. United States Food and Drug Administration regulation of clinical software in the era of artificial intelligence and machine learning. Mayo Clinic Proceedings: Digital Health. 2025;3(3):100231. https://doi.org/10.1016/j.mcpdig.2025.100231.
47. Singhal K, Tu T, Gottweis J, Sayres R, Wulczyn E, Amin M, Hou L, Clark K, Pfohl SR, Cole-Lewis H, Neal D, Rashid QM, Schaekermann M, Wang A, Dash D, Chen JH, Shah NH, Lachgar S, Mansfield PA, et al. Toward expert-level medical question answering with large language models. Nat Med. 2025;31(3):943–50. https://doi.org/10.1038/s41591-024-03423-7.
48. Tierney AA, Gayre G, Hoberman B, Mattern B, Ballesca M, Wilson Hannay SB, Castilla K, Lau CS, Kipnis P, Liu V, Lee K. Ambient artificial intelligence scribes: learnings after 1 year and over 2.5 million uses. NEJM Catalyst. 2025;6(5):CAT.25.0040. https://doi.org/10.1056/CAT.25.0040.
49. Ueda D, Walston SL, Matsumoto T, Deguchi R, Tatekawa H, Miki Y. Evaluating GPT-4-based ChatGPT's clinical potential on the NEJM quiz. BMC Digital Health. 2024;2(1):4. https://doi.org/10.1186/s44247-023-00058-5.
50. Vaswani A, Shazeer N, Parmar N, Uszkoreit J, Jones L, Gomez AN, Kaiser L, Polosukhin I. Attention is all you need (no. arXiv:1706.03762). arXiv. 2023; https://doi.org/10.48550/arXiv.1706.03762.
51. Wada A, Tanaka Y, Nishizawa M, Yamamoto A, Akashi T, Hagiwara A, Hayakawa Y, Kikuta J, Shimoji K, Sano K, Kamagata K, Nakanishi A, Aoki S. Retrieval-augmented generation elevates local LLM quality in radiology contrast media consultation. NPJ Digit Med. 2025;8:395. https://doi.org/10.1038/s41746-025-01802-z.

52. Wah JNK. Revolutionizing e-health: the transformative role of AI-powered hybrid chatbots in healthcare solutions. Front Public Health. 2025;13:1530799. https://doi.org/10.3389/fpubh.2025.1530799.
53. Wang H, Yang R, Alwakeel M, Kayastha A, Chowdhury A, Biro JM, Sorrentino AD, Handley JL, Hantzmon S, Bessias S, Economou-Zavlanos NJ, Bedoya A, Agrawal M, Ratwani RM, Poon EG, Pencina MJ, Pollak KI, Hong C. An evaluation framework for ambient digital scribing tools in clinical applications. Npj Digit Med. 2025;8(1):358. https://doi.org/10.1038/s41746-025-01622-1.
54. Webb E. How voice AI can slash healthcare clinicians' workloads—and offer companionship for older adults. Bus Insid. 2025; https://www.businessinsider.com/voice-ai-healthcare-admin-loneliness-companionship-2025-6.
55. Wendt SJ, Dinh CT, Sutcliffe M, Jones K, Scanlan JM, Smitherman JS. Deploying ambient clinical intelligence to improve care: a research article assessing the impact of nuance DAX on documentation burden and burnout. Future Healthc J. 2025:100450. https://doi.org/10.1016/j.fhj.2025.100450.
56. Wheeler CV. Regulating AI therapy Chatbots: a call for federal oversight. Texas A&M Law Rev. 2025;12(2):891–923. https://doi.org/10.37419/LR.V12.I2.9.
57. Woebot Health. Technically advanced. Responsible AI. Woebot Health. n.d. Retrieved August 14, 2025, from https://woebothealth.com/technology-overview/.
58. Wysa. Wysa for individuals | your AI companion for everyday wellbeing| AI based mental health platform. Wysa – Everyday Mental Health. n.d. Retrieved August 14, 2025, from https://www.wysa.com/for-individuals.
59. Yang R, Ning Y, Keppo E, Liu M, Hong C, Bitterman DS, Ong JCL, Ting DSW, Liu N. Retrieval-augmented generation for generative artificial intelligence in health care. Npj Health Syst. 2025;2(1):2. https://doi.org/10.1038/s44401-024-00004-1.
60. Youper. Youper: artificial intelligence for mental health. n.d. Retrieved August 14, 2025, from https://www.youper.ai/.
61. Zhang G, Xu Z, Jin Q, Chen F, Fang Y, Liu Y, Rousseau JF, Xu Z, Lu Z, Weng C, Peng Y. Leveraging long context in retrieval augmented language models for medical question answering. Npj Digit Med. 2025;8(1):239. https://doi.org/10.1038/s41746-025-01651-w.
62. Zhong W, Luo J, Zhang H. The therapeutic effectiveness of artificial intelligence-based chatbots in alleviation of depressive and anxiety symptoms in short-course treatments: A systematic review and meta-analysis. J Affect Disord. 2024;356:459–69. https://doi.org/10.1016/j.jad.2024.04.057.

Index

S. Scholz et al. (eds.), *Advancements in Digital Health and Care*,
https://doi.org/10.1007/978-3-032-16837-5

MIX
Papier aus verantwortungsvollen Quellen
Paper from responsible sources
FSC® C105338

If you have any concerns about our products,
you can contact us on
ProductSafety@springernature.com

In case Publisher is established outside the EU,
the EU authorized representative is:
Springer Nature Customer Service Center GmbH
Europaplatz 3, 69115 Heidelberg, Germany

Printed by Libri Plureos GmbH
in Hamburg, Germany